MODERN AND TRADITIONAL HEALTH CARE IN DEVELOPING SOCIETIES

Conflict and Co-operation

Edited by

Christine I. Zeichner, Ph.D.

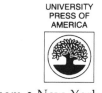

UNIVERSITY
PRESS OF
AMERICA

Lanham • New York • London

Copyright © 1988 by

University Press of America,® Inc.

4720 Boston Way
Lanham, MD 20706

3 Henrietta Street
London WC2E 8LU England

British Cataloging in Publication Information Available

Library of Congress Cataloging-in-Publication Data

Modern and traditional health care in developing societies : conflict
and co-operation / edited by Christiane I. Zeichner.
p. cm. Includes bibliographies.
1. Public health—Developing countries. 2. Medical care—
Developing countries. 3. Folk medicine—Developing countries.
4. Medical anthropology—Developing countries. I. Zeichner, Christiane I.
RA441.5.M63   1988
362.1'09172'4—dc 19   88–12138 CIP
ISBN 0–8191–6992–7 (alk. paper)
ISBN 0–8191–6993–5 (pbk. : alk. paper)

For
my husband Ben
my son Gregory and
my daughter Nicole

Acknowledgements

IN ACKNOWLEDGING MY DEBT TO OTHERS I WISH FIRST TO thank John H. Morgan who made this volume possible. My husband Ben Zeichner has been generous with his encouragement, assistance at each step, and most of all his critical talent.

I am most grateful to the National Institute of Health Education and Welfare and the Association of Indic-Islamic Studies for providing me with the opportunity and financial support to spend two months in Pakistan. This gave me a valuable firsthand view of medical systems in a developing society and intensive contact with those working in the health care field, especially in the area of health care modernization.

Likewise, I wish to thank all contributors for the fine quality of their work and for their willing co-operation. Finally, special recognition goes to the staff of University Press of America for their assistance and patience taking my numerous phone calls and their reviewer for the many valuable suggestions and commends.

Preface

THE DISSOLUTION OF COLONIAL POWER STRUCTURES IN the aftermath of World War II led to the emergence of new nations eager for the benefit of modern economic and medical technology. Their own interest in modernization, was soon paralleled by the Soviet Bloc's and the western world's interest in their problems. However, in spite continued economic aid for their social and economic progress by both superpowers and their allies, development in the field of health care remains far behind that of industrialized societies.

This volume addresses the major problem areas that contribute to poor health conditions in the third world: Poverty, poor sanitation, uneven distribution of health resources and services, suboptimal planning, poor management, and political instability. Its focus however, is on the conflict and cooperation between traditional health care systems and their modern counterparts. Despite an idealization of scientific medical knowledge and technology in the developing world, barriers exist that often prevent their direct application. These barriers usually reflect conflicting socio-cultural and political attitudes toward health modernization. Consequently, as scientific medical technology is used in modernization efforts, and as inter-systemic conflicts and disharmonies increase, the importance of understanding the traditional values of the people who live in the third world's rural areas grow more urgent.

Modernization goals and ideals of developing countries reflect those of their educated, politically articulate sector. The judgements that follow therefore, usually emanate from those leaders. Leaders' attitudes may not reflect those targeted for governmental health programs: the rural poor, whose perceptions and values will greatly determine the success of governmental health modernization policies. Conflict occurs, when indiginenous populations resist or create obstacles to modern health care approaches. Traditional leaders and healers then struggle to protect their own interests, and those of their people.

This area of study is insufficiently recognized in the health literature, owing to national disillusionment with the politics of developing societies. But with tensions mounting economically, socially and politically in developing countries across the world—any of them easily reached in less than 24 hours by plane—this inquiry becomes a timely subject.

This volume contains 18 original, previously unpublished essays drawn on a variety of disciplines. They are compiled by a sociologist and written by academics who as anthropologists, physicians, psychologists, public health professionals, and sociologists recently conducted field research on various health care problems in Africa, South America, the Carribean, Asia and the Middle East.

The organization of the material is in three major sections. **Section I,** focuses on the co-existence and competition of modern scientific medicine with its traditional counterpart. Perry offers a broad overview of how mortality and morbidity, uneven distribution of health resources and services, and suboptimal planning and management all contribute to poor health conditions in developing societies. B. Zeichner's piece on psychiatry in the People's Republic of China, shows how harmoniously this country merges the old with the new. Traditional Chinese medical approaches are taught both in general medical schools and in traditional medical schools. He shows how the People's Republic of China attempts her own unique synthesis of traditional and modern psychiatric care. In contrast Tsai reveals the growing conflict between traditional Chinese practitioners and western trained counterparts in Taiwan. He argues, that industrialization, economic growth and its subsequent socio-economic effects have turned people away from things traditional, to avoid allegations of "backwardness". None of the 30 medical schools in Taiwan today provide training in traditional Chinese medicine. Traditional Chinese medicine in Taiwan is offered only in small, private hospitals and clinics. The large government-operated public hospitals do not employ traditional treatment approaches, except acupuncture. Tsai identifies as a serious problem, the lack of government imposed controls on the pharmaceutic industry and licensure. This situation brings about widespread abuse of prescription drugs and foments disharmony between modern medical pratitioners and those who dispense medications.

The piece by Allman expands the idea of co-operation between traditional and modern health care approaches. She discusses how the Haitian Division of Family Hygiene trains indigenous mid-wives to assist in the deliveries of rural Haitian women, to improve childbirth practices. Traditional birthing is described. Conflict between the two medical approaches is also reported by Davis, who points to Morocco's rural population's dissatisfaction with modern medicine. Identified are factors such as high cost, inconvenient clinic locations, lack of courtesy and social distance. Patients of humble origins felt more comfortable with healers of their own gender, and who are closer to their own social class and culture.

C. Zeichner examines family planning in Pakistan, where implementation of family planning programs has advanced knowledge of communication, cummunity involvement and motivation of target couples. She discusses obstacles to the development of birth controlled population planning.

Pieces by Fosu, Harvey, Willard and LaDue concentrate on the type of agents that are thought to cause disease. Widespread throughout the world are some five basic categories of events or situations which in folk etiology, are believed to be responsible for illness.

These are sorcery, breach of taboo, loss of soul, intrusion of a disease causing spirit, and intrusion of a disease object. Not

every society recognizes all five categories; indeed many
groups are selective in the emphasis placed upon one or a
combination of causes. Fosu, in his study of how a traditional
rural Ghanaian community views health and diseases, finds
causes of disease be they natural or supernatural ones, to be
most important aspects of therapy. The younger better educated with new economic opportunities and more contact with
urban communities show a modern scientific attitude toward
illness, and reject the idea that diseases are caused supernaturally.

This idea is confirmed by Harvey, who suggests that a
group's heritage is important to remember when making policy decisions about modern medical development. Haiti and
Cuba, are largely populated by peoples of African ancestry
and voodoo is thus an important part of their traditional
medicine.

The process of health modernization must be a gradual,
transitional one, that respects the outlooks and perspectives of
these rural people.

Willard's piece is the only one included in this volume that
covers health care in the United States. It is an illustration of
how traditional and modern health care can co-exist in harmony among sub-groups of an advanced, industrialized nation. He discusses possible advantages and methods of
integrating Shamanism, practiced by American Indian healers, into modern health care programs for American Indian
cultures.

Section II, deals with substantive issues of public health
and traditional beliefs. The thrust of Lambrecht's two essays is
that human culture and behavior play important roles in the
spread and distribution of disease. He points out that large-
scale water impoundment and irrigation development operations in tropical countries have spread parasitic diseases. He
suggests that improved sanitation would greatly reduce man
made tick, snail and mosquito breeding sites and reduce
disease transmission.

Seller and Wise analyze malnutrition. Sellers argues that

due to protein-energy malnutrition most children among less privileged populations of underdeveloped nations show retarded growth and impaired mental development by the time they reach school age. Wise reports his research in Guatemala with Incaparina a low cost, high protein mixture of vegetable sources, widely expected to help reduce malnutrition. The last piece in this section is by Frenk, who discusses medical modernization via state intervention in Mexico.

Section III contains four essays that examine the interaction between political ideology, armed conflict and health care delivery. In addition to the factors mentioned in the two above sections, health care systems and patterns of medical development of poor nations are influenced by the political alignments they make. Foreign aid may either be requested from communist powers or the free western world. Oris's essay on Cuban health care shows how countries under communist influence may apply soviet methods of planning for medical development, while those aligned with the western bloc may adopt western methods.

The politicization of health campaigns in civil war torn third world countries is common. In his essay on malaria control activities in Nicaragua, Garfield reports that resistance to accepting anti-malaria medication comes from both pro-communist as well as pro-western groups, each accusing the other of spying while providing malaria case detection and treatment.

The two last papers in this section by Dagher, Bashshur, Kronfol and Haydar deal with health care activities in Lebanon, a country of 3 million people in the shadows of civil war and foreign occupation. Lebanon's large number of casualties and refugees have drastically affected health care delivery and priorities. Medical attention is mainly limited to the wounded rather than to those with chronic diseases.

C.I.Z.

THE EDITOR

Christiane I. Zeichner received her B.A. from the George Washington University in Washington D.C., an M.S.W. from The Catholic University of America, School of Social Service, Washington, D.C. and a Ph.D. in sociology from American University in Washington, D.C. She is on the staff of the Department of Health and Human Services, Bureau of Forensic Psychiatry, and on the faculty of the Department of Sociology, at American University, both in Washington, D.C. She has held faculty appointments at Virginia Commonwealth University, Richmond, Virginia and The Catholic University of America, Washington, D.C. Among the many grants she has received, the most recent one is from the National Institute of Health Education and Welfare and the Association of Indic Islamic Studies, to spend time in Pakistan to pursue her research interests in the field of health care modernization.

CONTRIBUTORS

(NOTE: Contributors are listed in alphabetical order. When a chapter is co-authored, the first author is listed alphabetically and the co-authors are listed alphabetically immediately under the first author).

Allman, Suzanne received her Ph.D. in anthropological linguistics from the University of Aix-Marseille, France.

Bashshur, Rashid received his Ph.D. in sociology from the University of Michigan, Ann Arbor, Michigan.

Kronfol, Nabil received his M.D. and Dr.P.H. from Harvard University, Cambridge, Massachusetts.

Abu Haydar, Elizabeth received her M.P.H. from the University of Michigan and her Ph.D. from the School of Public Health, of the University of North Carolina, Chapel Hill, North Carolina.

Dagher, Fuad J. received his M.D. from the American University of Beirut, School of Medicine, Beirut, Lebanon.

Fosu, Gabriel B. received his Ph.D. in sociology from Brown University, Providence, Rhode Island.

Frenk, Julio received his M.D. from the National University of Mexico, Mexico City, Mexico, and an M.P.H. and Ph.D. in sociology from the University of Michigan, Ann Arbor, Michigan.

Garfield, Richard received his Dr.P.H. from Columbia University, School of Public Health, in New York City, New York.

Harvey, William B. received his Ph.D. in Education from North Carolina State University in Raleigh, North Carolina.

Lambrecht, Frank L. received an M.A. in biology and a Diploma of Tropical Medicine and Hygiene (D.T.M.H.) from the Tropical Institute of Antwerp, Belgium.

Orris, Peter received his M.D. from the University of Chicago Medical School and an M.P.H. from Yale University, School of Public Health, New Haven Connecticut.

Perry, Henry B. received his M.D., M.P.H. and a Ph.D. in sociology from Johns Hopkins University, Baltimore Maryland.

Schaefer-Davis, Susan received her Ph.D. in anthropology from the University of Michigan, Ann Arbor, Michigan.

Sellers, Stephen G. received his Ph.D. in anthropology from Brandeis University, Waltham, Massachusetts.

Tsai, Wen-Hui received his Ph.D. from the University of California, at Berkeley, California.

Willard, William received his Ph.D. anthropology from the University of Arizona, Tucson, Arizona.

LaDue, Robin A. received her Ph.D. in psychology from the Washington State University, Pullman, Washington.

Wise, Robert P. received his M.D. from Northwestern University, Medical School and an M.P.H. from Harvard School of Public Health, Cambridge, Massachusetts.

Zeichner, Ben received his M.D. from New York University, School of Medicine, New York City, New York.

Contents

Modern and Traditional Health Care Delivery: A Problem of Choice

CHAPTER 1

Health in the Developing World: An Overview of Obstacles and Opportunities

Henry B. Perry, III

Health conditions in the developing world still lag substantially behind those in the developed world. Poverty, uneven distribution of health resources and services, and suboptimal planning and management all contribute to poor health conditions. Improvement of health conditions will depend upon the most effective possible use of scarce resources in programs of scientifically proven effectiveness toward the most frequent and serious health problems. Non-physician personnel, backup support for primary care workers, local financing, and community participation all appear to be essential to improving health conditions in the developing world.

THIS CHAPTER ADDRESSES BRIEFLY FOUR MAJOR problem areas related to health care in the developing world. The first is the health status of persons living in the developing world and their particular causes of morbidity. Secondly, there is the problem of poverty, its effect on health status, and the lack of

3

funds for development of health services. Thirdly, there exists the problem of uneven distribution of existing health resources and services. Finally, there is the problem of inadequate management resulting in ineffective and inefficient use of existing resources. Approaches to improving the provision of health services and, more importantly, to actually improving the health status of persons in the developing world are considered as well.

While this chapter focuses upon technical problems related to improving health in the developing world, it should be recognized that behind all of these technical issues are profound social, political, and economic problems which make the resolution of the identified problems so difficult. As Rohde observes (1984:42), "professionalism, international health bureaucracies, and social power structures all combine in a strange political *melange* to ignore or even impede progress toward child survival."

Mortality and Morbidity in the Developing World

In the developing world the average life expectancy at birth is 53 years, almost twenty years less than the 70.3 years of life expectancy enjoyed by persons in the developed world. One-tenth of the life of the average person in the developing world is disrupted by ill health. Infant mortality rates and mortality rates for children under 5 years of age in low-income countries are 10–20 times higher than those observed in developed countries. In many areas of developing countries, one-third to one-half of all children die before reaching the age of five. In many developing countries, half of all the deaths in the population are in children under five. Once reaching age five, however, a child's life expectancy is only 6–8 years less than that for a child living in a developed country (Evans et al., 1981); World Bank, 1980)

There are two major causes of morbidity and mortality in the developing world: fecally-transmitted diseases and airborne diseases. The most common fecally-transmitted disease is infectious diarrhea. The World Health Organization (1980) has estimated that more than 750 million children under five years of age in the developing world develop acute diarrhea each year and that 3–6 million persons die from dehydration caused by acute diarrhea. Eighty percent of these deaths are in children less than two years of age.

Other important fecally transmitted diseases are polio, typhoid, and cholera along with intestinal parasites. An estimated 650 million persons are infected with ascaris (roundworms), 450 million with ancylostomiasis (hookworms), 350 million with amebiasis, and 350 million with trichuriasis (whipworm).

A variety of airborne diseases are encountered in the developing world. Among the most important are tuberculosis, pneumonia, measles, and influenza. Other airborne diseases of significance are diphtheria, bronchitis, whooping cough, meningitis, and chicken pox.

Particularly in children, lowered immunity brought about by malnutrition results in much higher mortality rates from the above illnesses and others than would be observed among well-nourished children. Over seventy percent of deaths among Latin American children less than five but beyond the perinatal period were due to fecally related diseases, airborne disease (including measles), or malnutrition (World Bank, 1980). Even in very poor areas of the Third World, well-nourished children have mortality rates similar to those of children in the developed world, while malnourished children die at much higher rates (Rohde, 1984).

Although the average life expectancy has been increasing in the developing world, there is recent evidence that this rate is slowing. Whereas between 1950 and 1960 the average annual rate of increase was 0.64 years, this had fallen to 0.40 years fifteen years later (Evans et al, 1981).

Poverty: Its Impact upon Health Status
and Financing of Health Services

The important influence of a population's standard of living upon health status has been exemplified by historical studies demonstrating major improvements in incidence of mortality from cholera, typhoid fever, and tuberculosis prior to the availability of effective specific treatments.

Poverty in developing countries, associated with rapid population growth, inadequate nutrition, as well as crowded and unsanitary living conditions, is a major cause of morbidity and mortality. The overriding constraint in imposing health conditions in low-income countries is the extreme poverty of much of the population, frequently with per capita incomes of less than $250, and the low level of the gross national product per capita, less than $500 per capita in 53 developing countries (World Bank, 1980). The ability of the people themselves or their governments to finance health services is thus extremely limited.

Current estimates are that by the year 1990, public expenditures for health will average about US $3 per capita in low-income countries. "Predictions for the year 2000", Evans et al note (1981:1122), "show little further improvement, particularly in the low-income countries, with the gap between rich and poor countries continuing to widen."

Uneven Distribution of Health Resources and Services

It is estimated that 85% of the developing world's rural population lacks access to even basic medical services (Mejia, et al, 1978). The physician-population ratios in the urban areas of developing countries approximate those for the developed world (1:500 to 1:2,000) whereas in rural areas these ratios are in the order of 1:10,000 to 1:200,000. Thus there are 5 to 200 times more persons per physician in rural areas than in urban areas of developing countries (Perry and Breitner, 1982). Hospitals utilizing expensive advanced technology can be found in almost all major cities of developing countries. In many countries, two-thirds of the government's health budget is devoted to urban medical education and the related costs of urban teaching hospitals (World Bank, 1980).

One of the consequences of an emphasis upon advanced hospital care and urban medical education has been the development of an "hour-glass" distribution of health personnel, with a relatively large number of physicians at the top, a relatively large number of indigenous practitioners at the bottom, and relatively few health personnel in between. The lack of supporting personnel has led to inefficiency in the provision of health services. The emphasis upon advanced hospital care and the education of physicians has also produced an overemphasis upon curative services and a lack of attention to preventive health services.

In rural areas, sparsely distributed health facilities have left most of the population without access to basic services. Studies have indicated that the utilization of rural health facilities diminishes abruptly for persons who live more than 3–5 kilometers away from a health facility (World Bank, 1980, Jolly and King, 1966).

Suboptimal Planning and Management

It has been repeatedly observed that the existing health resources in developing countries, even though they are quite limited, are frequently not utilized to their potential. Perhaps the major conclusion of the World Bank's Health Sector policy paper (1980:7) was the following:

> It is now evident that the most persistent problems in improving health do not result from the complexity of medical technology and only partially from the scarcity of financial resources; rather, they derive principally from problems in the design and implementation of policy, management, and logistics.

There are two components of the problem of planning and management. First of all, the capability to plan and implement programs which make the best use of limited resources is inadequate in most developing countries. Secondly, planning and management is frequently concentrated in central Ministry offices among persons who have an inadequate understanding of the real constraints on implementation at the operating level (Evans et al, 1981).

One particular weakness in planning and management activities noted by Evans is at the district level:

> The weakest link in the administrative chain of most developing countries are institutions at district and local levels, which are usually poorly staffed, have inadequate authority or control of resources and are unable to provide the necessary support and supervision of field staff. The development of planning and administrative capacity at the district level is of special importance, since this is normally the lowest tier of the health services organization still communicating directly with the central government unit also in contact with the villages, aware of their needs, and in a position to encourage community participation (Evans et al, 1981).

One aspect of planning and management of critical importance, but which is usually seriously deficient, is that pertaining to the supply of drugs and vaccines. In many developing countries, drugs constitute 40–60% of the health budget (versus 15–20% in developed countries) and are the major source of private health expenditures. Poor planning frequently results in a shortage (or absence) of essential drugs. Inappropriate prescription practices for available drugs is common. Furthermore, "public health planners", writes Cross (1981:209) "are sometimes surprised at how much even the poorest individuals will pay for overpriced or marginally useful medicines sold at local pharmacies and shops." It has been shown in selected cases that a savings of between 25% and 70% of the expenses for drugs can be achieved by limiting the availability of nonessential drugs, by bulk purchasing, by promoting generic alternatives, and by introducing controls against overprescription (Evans et al, 1981). In developing countries, deficiencies in policy formulation, management, and logistics are particularly serious because of the high incidence of disease and death and because of the scarcity of resources available to reduce disease and death.

Possible Solutions

As a result of the declaration of "Health for All by the Year 2000" at the Alma-Ata Conference on Primary Health Care sponsored by the World Health Organization and UNICEF in 1978 (WHO, 1978), interest in the extension of basic health services throughout the world has increased greatly. There have arisen six major strategies related to the extension of health services that are now thought to have a maximum potential impact on morbidity and mortality in the developing world.

First and foremost is an emphasis upon the development of low-cost preventive and curative services of scientifically proven effectiveness aimed at the most common and serious diseases. Secondly, is an emphasis upon the utilization of non-physician midlevel health personnel and village health workers in the provision of these primary care services. Thirdly, is an emphasis upon the development of a backup system of supervision and support for primary care workers. Fourth, is an emphasis upon new forms of financing health programs, especially from the private sector. Fifth, is an emphasis upon community involvement in the design and implementation of health programs. Rigorous evaluation and monitoring of health programs constitutes the sixth emphasis in improving health services.

Effective Low Cost Services

Gwatkin et al (1980) recently reviewed the results of ten health projects throughout the developing world and concluded that:

In the hands of able leaders and in populations of up to
60,000–70,000, well-designed and effectively operated
projects can reduce infant and child mortality rates by one
third to one half or more within one to five years, at a cost
of less than the equivalent of 2 percent of per capita
income—an amount no greater than that currently being
allocated to health nationally.

Berggren et al (1981), showed that for $1.60 per person per
year, mortality rates in Haiti could be lowered by more than
two-thirds.

What are the factors responsible for the success of these
activities? Gwatkin et al (1980:18, 24) listed the general components common to these programs:

a) widespread coverage
b) nutrition monitoring
c) reliance upon village-based non-physician personnel
d) maternal immunization against tetanus
e) targeted nutritional supplementation for pregnant
   women and malnourished children
f) effective training programs
g) leadership and organizational effectiveness

Among the specific health care activities of importance, those
developed by Berggren et al (1981) are worthy of discussion:

a) lessons in health and nutrition (15 minute talks for
   adults on such topics as breast feeding, frequency and
   content of child feeding, method of oral rehydration,
   and use of the 'road to health' growth chart)
b) targeted supplemental feedings or referral to local nutritional rehabilitation centers for children with third
   degree malnutrition or weight loss
c) demonstration nutrition education for mothers
d) demonstration of oral rehydration for mothers and
   health personnel
e) screening and treatment of tuberculosis
f) deworming with piperazine (primarily to stimulate interest of mothers in the health program)
g) immunizations (DPT, polio, measles, tetanus, BCG)

h) support of traditional birth attendants (classes, provision of kits for care of umbilical cord)

These general and specific approaches developed in successful health programs are likely to produce the greatest impacts in lowering mortality and morbidity at minimum cost.

Utilization of Non-Physician Personnel

The second major point of emphasis in approaching health problems in the developing world is the utilization of non-physician midlevel health personnel and village health worker personnel as providers of primary care (Storms, 1979). The scarcity of physicians in rural areas of the developing world necessitates the development of roles for them which maximize their training and skills. Furthermore, experience in developing countries as well as in the United States has strongly supported the idea that, with proper training and supervision, non-physician personnel can provide high quality primary care services (Perry and Breitner, 1982). Thus the physician's role is more properly viewed as a supervisor and backup support person for the primary health care provider. Flahault, (1978:129) notes that,

> "as the developed and developing countries alike have grappled with the shortage of medical manpower, they have increasingly come to realize that much of the problem is attributable to the inefficient use of physician's time."

In recognition of these needs, there has arisen a great interest in midlevel health personnel and in voluntary village health workers as providers of primary care. The village health worker is generally a lifelong resident of the village he or she serves and is usually selected by his follow villagers to receive a training of four to six weeks in length. Their training emphasizes preventive health measures such as vaccinations, identification of malnourished children, nutrition education, curative health measures such as treatment of diarrhea with oral rehydration fluid and antibiotic treatment of respiratory infections, first aid, and referral of patients to a health center or hospital when indicated (Arole, 1973).

Increasing importance is being given to an adequately prepared midlevel health worker with skills to function as a primary care provider (Smith, 1978). The traditional auxiliary with six months of training is now viewed as inadequately prepared for this type of role. An 18–24 month period of training in primary care activities qualifies this person to function as a teacher and supervisor of village health workers. (Flahault, 1978; Perry and Breitner, 1982). Such persons are ideally mature leaders selected from the area they are to serve prior to beginning their training.

Backup Support for Primary Care Workers

The third major need in the development of health care programs is an emphasis upon backup systems for support of primary care activities at the village level (World Bank, 1980). A general dictum has evolved which states that the less training a health worker has received, the more supervision that person requires (Flahault, 1978). Thus, the village health worker requires a great deal of supervision if he or she is to be effective and maintain interest in the role. Since such persons are usually voluntary (and hence less committed to their work than paid employees), backup support in the form of supervision and provision of essential drugs and supplies is most important (World Bank, 1980:46). The importance of backup support systems has also been emphasized by Wray (in Storms, 1978):

> "No matter how well-intentioned the program, no matter how adequate or inadequate the training, unless auxiliaries (including village health workers) are part of a system that is capable of providing them with satisfactory guidance when needed, the necessary supplies and equipment to carry out the tasks assigned them, and a referral system to

which they can send problems with which they cannot deal, they are not likely to be able to function effectively."

Midlevel health personnel clearly have a most important role to play in the backup and field supervision of village health workers. These midlevel health personnel also need backup and supervision themselves. The availability of physicians with sufficient training in primary care to perform this role is quite important but usually lacking. In addition, the availability of physicians and hospital services for patients requiring hospitalization and possibly surgery are an essential ingredient for effective backup support. Too often, however, hospital backup support is simply unavailable.

Although surgery is not a primary care activity, it is nevertheless quite important as a supportive function for primary care workers. By virtue of expanding access to primary care services, greater needs for surgical support services will arise. As noted by Dr. Halfdan Mahler, Director General of the World Health organization, (1980:12):

> "people in need must have access to skilled surgical care at first line referral hospitals . . . Yet although these are high priority matters for everybody, the vast majority of the world's population has no access whatsoever to skilled surgical care and little is being done to find a solution. In too many countries, even if people living in capital cities have access to surgical care, most of the population who live outside these cities do not."

Such systems of referral care and supervision are part of the "district" approach to the development of regionalized health care delivery programs. Such an approach places planning and administration at the district level for populations in the range of 100,000 to 500,000 persons. The need to implement and document the effectiveness of programs at this level is viewed by Gwatkin and his colleagues (1980) as a very important priority at this time. It is now clear that well-designed and well-administered small scale programs serving 10–60,000 persons can be quite effective in lowering mortality rates. For the larger scale projects, however, a much greater degree of organizational coordination is required.

> "Means will have to be found to reconcile the degree of centralized organization and leadership necessary for the implementation of large-scale efforts with the full local participation and responsibility that are essential to equitable programs" (Gwatkins et al, 1980:32).

The need at present is for programs developed at the district level which incorporate community input into the planning and management process and are based upon a systematic regionalized approach to health care delivery. An integral part of this approach is the development of a simple information system which will allow program administrators to assess the effectiveness of their activities.

Local Private Financing

The fourth point of emphasis in developing health care programs is the need for alternative private methods of financing health services. As one authority on health care financing concluded,

> "general tax revenues and social insurance funds, although they are the major sources of health care support, are not likely to suffice if developing countries want to achieve universal access to health care in the forseeable future . . . Most developing countries will thus have to rely on a variety of private sector sources of support in their efforts to expand and improve health care more rapidly" (Zschock, 1979:27).

In previous decades there has developed the attitude that the financing of health programs for the poor is the responsibility of government. Such an idea is no longer tenable for three reasons. First of all, it is becoming increasingly clear that the governments of low-income countries will not have the necessary resources to finance low-cost health services for their entire population without a major shift of funds from other sectors to the health sector. This is viewed as highly unlikely. Secondly, it is now recognized that families spend at least as much, or perhaps more, per capita on health care than do most governments in low-income countries (Evans et al, 1981). Most of these family expenditures are either for drugs or for traditional healers. Thus even the poor have the capability of bearing a major portion of the cost of inexpensive health programs. Thirdly, it is now appreciated that a dependence upon private financing results in greater attention of the program to local concerns and also to greater community participation (Gwatkins et al, 1980). Thus, as the World Bank (1980:46) concluded, "local financing also generally strengthens the accountability of the system to its clients." Strong incentives to minimize waste and inefficiency are created which too often are absent in health programs totally supported by the public sector.

It is the policy of government health programs in many areas to make drugs available at no charge. As O'Connor (1981:20) states,

> "the cost of "free" drugs is scarcity, stock-out, and disillusionment. Ministry of Health staff are dispirited by trying to provide services without resources, and the people are frustrated by receiving so much less than promised . . . A realistic solution may lie in the development of a creative partnership between government responsibility to organize the supply of basic pharmaceuticals and individual responsibility to pay for what is needed and valued."

In China, one of the few low-income countries with widespread health services, the health station at the community level is totally self-supported as is the lowest-level hospital. General tax revenues are used to support secondary and tertiary hospitals as well as nationwide preventive health campaigns (Zschock, 1979). The need now in the developing world is for private financing schemes from the widest spectrum of alternative sources . . . "ensuring that these resources are a net addition to public funding rather than a substitute for it" (Evans et al, 1981:1123).

Community Participation

The fifth point of emphasis in the development of low-cost health programs is community participation in the design and implementation of health programs (WHO, 1978:23,). In the words of a WHO Expert Committee, lasting results in rural health care "can be achieved only through active community participation" (WHO, 1979:13). Community participation encourages local initiative and responsibility.

After a personal review of a large number of health programs in Latin America, Werner (1976) classified programs into two types: community supportive and community oppressive. "Community supportive" programs encourage local decision-making and self-reliance while "community oppressive" programs are paternalistic and encourage greater dependency and unquestioning acceptance of outside roles and decisions. Werner also noted that "community supportive" programs were usually small and private while "community oppressive" programs were large regional or national programs. This led Werner to conclude that the most important question concerning rural health care today is, "how can the people-supportive features of outstanding small, non-government pilot projects be adapted for regional or country-wide outreach" (Werner, 1976:7)?

By facilitating community self-reliance and responsibility in the selection of village health workers and organization of their work by village development committees, for instance, the capability of the community to focus its efforts on other priority areas outside of health is thus enhanced, thereby promoting the process of socio-economic development. The methodology of this approach within the context of large-scale programs has yet to be worked out, particularly in the selection of community representatives and their participation in planning and policy formulation at the district level.

Evaluation

Having now discussed five points of emphasis in improving health care in low-income countries, we now turn to the sixth and final point: evaluation and monitoring of programs. Gwatkin et al (1980:33) are quite emphatic in their insistence upon the inclusion of a rigorous evaluation of the costs and mortality impact in large-scale health programs:

> "The current prospect is that increasing numbers of large-scale primary health and nutrition care projects will be initiated during the years immediately ahead . . . Over-enthusiastic, unreflective implementation runs the danger of inflicting serious harm on a fragile, imcompletely under-stood idea. This gives a particular urgency to evaluation efforts to monitor the progress of large-scale primary care programs and to provide early warning at the first sign of any failure of primary care approaches to live up to their potential."

Firm evidence indicating the impact of such programs on mortality and their associated costs will be necessary if a strong case for investment in health care can be continued to be made in the future.

In addition, simple program-management information systems are needed if program administrators are to be able to monitor the ongoing effectiveness of the progress of the program and make necessary changes quickly. Such information is also needed in assessing the cost of program activities. Thus, information systems are vital for maximizing program effectiveness as well as for completing a cost-benefit evaluation.

In conclusion, attaining the goal of health for all by the year 2000 will require the implementation of innovative approaches in maximizing the health benefit at a minimum cost. The points of emphasis in program development which have been discussed above will no doubt be supplemented by new philosophies and technologies during the coming decades. Nevertheless, the lessons from recent experiences are sufficiently clear to provide adequate and effective sign posts for the present in extending health services in the developing world.

As biomedical scientific research advances our knowledge of effective low-cost techniques for preventing or treating common serious diseases throughout the developing world, the sociological and anthropological issues of implementing these effective technologies will assume an ever growing importance. Understanding how to best mobilize available political, financial, and manpower resources into a process of health care delivery which uses these new low-cost technologies constitutes a major task for the behavioral sciences in the coming decades. The challenge is to "learn how to implement mass programs for needy people in villages throughout the world" (Taylor et al, 1983).

References

Arole, M. (1978) "Village Health Workers and Community Involvement in Health Care Delivery in India."
In Ronald W. McNeur, (ed.). *The Changing Roles and Education of Health Care Personnel Worldwide in View of the Increase of Basic Health Services*. Philadelphia: Society for Health and Human Values.

Berggren, W. L., D. C. (Eubank), G. G. Berggren (1981) "Reduction of Mortality in Rural Haiti Through a Primary Health Care Program." *New England Journal of Medicine*. 304:1324–1330.

Cross, P. "Who Will Pay: Financing Drug Supplies." (1981) In J. D. Quick (ed.). *Managing Drug Supply*. Boston: Management Sciences for Health.

Evans, J. R., K. L. Hall, and J. Warford (1981) "Shattuck Lecture-Health Care in the Developing World: Problems of Scarcity and Choice." *New England Journal of Medicine*. 305:1117–1127.

Flahault, D. (1978) "Primary Health Care by Non-Physicians." In A. Mejia, T. L. Hall, and E. Royston, (eds.). *Health Manpower Planning*. Geneva: WHO. 177–200.

Gwatkins, D. R., J. R. Wilcox, and J. D. Wray (1980) *Can Health and Nutrition Interventions Make a Difference?* Washington, D. C.: Overseas Development Council, Monograph No. 13.

Jolly, R. and M. King (1966) "The Organization of Health Services." In M. King (ed.). *Medical Care in Developing Countries*. Nairobi: Oxford University Press.

Mahler, H. (1981) "Surgery and Health for All." Mexico City: Address to the Biennial Congress of the International College of Surgeons.

Majia, A., T. L. Hall, and E. Royston (1978) "Manpower Distribution." In T. L. Hall and A. Majia, (eds.). *Health Manpower Planning*. Geneva: WHO, pp. 147–176.

O'Connor, R. (1981) "The Dimensions of Drug Supply." In J. D. Quick (ed.), *Managing Drug Supply*. Boston: Management Sciences for Health.

Perry, H. B. and B. Breitner (1982) *Physician Assistants: Their Contribution to Health Care*. New York: Human Sciences Press.

Rohde, Jon E. (1984) "Why the Other Half Dies. The Science and Politics of Child Mortality in the Third World." *Les Carnets de L'enfance, 61/62, A Child Survival and Development Revolution*. Geneva: UNESCO, pp. 35–67.

Smith, R. A. (1978) "Designing an Appropriate Approach to Improved Health Service Coverage." In R. A. Smith (ed.). *Manpower and Primary Health Care: Guidelines for Improving/ Extending Health Services in Developing Countries*. Honolulu: University Press of Hawaii.

Storms, D. (1979) *Training and Use of Auxiliary Health Workers: Lessons from Developing Countries*. Washington, D. C.: American Public Health Association, International Health Programs Monograph Series No. 3.

Taylor, C. E., R. S. S. Sarma, Robert L. Parket, et al (1983) *Child and Maternal Health Services in Rural India, the Narangwal Experiment, Volume I: Integrated Family Planning and Health Care*. Baltimore: Johns Hopkins University Press.

Werner, D. (1976) "Health Care and Human Dignity: A Subjective Look at Community-Based Rural Health Programs in Latin America." Palo Alto, California: Hesperian Foundation.

World Bank (1980) *Health Sector Policy Paper*. Washington, D. C.: World Bank

WHO (World Health Organization) *Primary Health Care: Report of the International Conference on Primary Health Care, Alma-Ata, USSR*. (1978) Geneva: World Health Organization. *Training and Utilization of Auxiliary Personnel for Rural Health Teams in Developing Countries*. (1979) Geneva; Technical Report Series 633. *Sixth Report on the World Health Situation, Part Two: Review by Country and Area*. (1980) Geneva; World Health Organization.

Zschock, D. K. (1979) *Health Care Financing in Developing Countries*. Washington, D. C.: American Public Health Association, International Health Monograph Series No. 1.

CHAPTER 2

Modern and Traditional Psychiatry in the People's Republic of China

Ben Zeichner

China provides an illustration of a country with an organized system of medical theory and practice in continuous operation for almost three thousand years. Western medical and psychiatric concepts were introduced into China at the turn of this century. Following the communist revolution, soviet psychiatric methods gained influence. Currently, China is attempting her own synthesis of traditional chinese psychiatric concepts with western biological psychiatric approaches.

Introduction

CHINA IS A COUNTRY WITH A PARTICULARLY INTERESTING health system, for she has officially maintained her old indigenous science of traditional medicine alongside a functioning western system of medicine which entered China at the end of the last century.

Psychiatry, the diagnosis and treatment of emotional and behavioral disorders, is influenced by a society's view of man and his place in society. Thus in China psychiatry has reflected the social, scientific, and political changes of her long history, influences of the West, of the Soviet Union, and those of modern technology, while always preserving ideas of group and family allegiance. Today one finds in chinese psychiatry, a combination of modern western drugs, traditional chinese methods, and diagnostic categories such as "sexual nonconformity" unknown in the West (Wilson 1983).

Psychiatry in Traditional Chinese Medicine Before the Modern Era

Psychiatry in China has had a long history.

As in the West, in China it has passed through stages of naturalistic, religious, somatic, and psychological conceptualization.

Chinese medicine evolved in relative isolation, preserving written records from various dynasties over the past twenty five centuries (Tseng 1973). Earliest records concerning mental illness are found in the bone oracle inscriptions of the fourteenth century B.C., attributing headaches to the winds of the Yellow River Valley (Berman 1968). Cave paintings of greater antiquity depict the use of acupuncture needles. References to mania, confusion, depression, paranoia, and emotional stress are found in writings from three hundred B.C. (Liu 1981).

Eventually reknowned physicians codified medical knowledge, establishing principles of health and illness based upon ideas of natural harmonies and balanced forces whose proper relationships insured good health (Liu 1981; Tseng: 1973:).

As more precise anatomical knowledge grew, medical thought considered the roles of bodily organs in health maintenance, charging each organ with a specific function. Emotions were believed to arise from different organs as the flow of vital air through the body activated them. Harmonious living kept the currents flowing properly. Mental symptoms, "crazy talking", epilepsy, and hallucinations, were described in texts and related to fevers and to other disharmonies.

Classifications of mental illness expanded over the centuries. By the seventeenth century Wang Ketang had divided psychoses into three categories, each with and without excitation, and restlessness into nine categories, and panics into five categories. Unfortunately, these categories were never modified and treatments remained based upon their fixed classification, and upon earlier unmodified theories of polarity and disharmony.

By the end of the nineteenth century many conditions had been noted, and attention given to psychosomatic causation, and frustrated sexual desire, which somewhat paralleled western ideas of neurasthenia. The major treatment for psychiatric conditions, however, remained the use of ancient herbs, and the placement of acupuncture needles in specific skin sites thought to be portals of vital forces. Psychiatry remained an aspect of general medicine with no special books, facilities or training, but this was soon to change.

The Modern Era: Psychiatry Before
Mao Tse Tung

As China came under western influence at the end of the last century, traditional medicine suffered a loss in prestige and began to decline (Taipale 1973). Most mental patients remained in the care of relatives, of non psychiatric doctors, or were left to fend for themselves. Now, however efforts to establish mental hospitals began.

Following the demise of small short lived institutions in Faitham and Hong Kong, Dr. John Kerr of the U.S. in 1897 established a hospital in Canton of 30 beds for mental and nervous disorders which survived for 40 years. By the nineteen thirties, efforts of american physicians Drs. A.H. Woods in Peking and R.S. Lyman in Shanghai led to the addition of psychiatric teaching to westernized medical schools and to the enlargement of psychiatric facilities. Most important Fanny Halpern of the University of Vienna developed numerous mental health organizations in Shanghai which lasted until the japanese occupation of World War Two (Koran 1972), Berman 1968).

After World War II, in an effort to obtain epidemiological data, the World Health Organization sent the american professor, Dr. Karl Bowman to Nationalist China to help found the National Neuropsychiatric Institute. Following his three month fact gathering stay in 1947, he reported that China, with more than 450 million people, had less than 50 psychiatrists, and that of the 50 medical schools only a few offered any instruction in psychiatry at all (Bermann 1968). Clearly, despite the introduction of western psychiatric ideas in certain selected centers, the treatment of the mentally ill was still rather primitive by western standards.

Psychiatry in the People's Republic of China 1949–1965:

The Influence of Mao Tse Tung

In 1949, following Mao Tse Tung's communist liberation of China, american and european psychiatric influence declined, and the psychodynamically oriented model of mental illness was abandoned as reflecting the now rejected bourgeois capitalistic view of man. Mao's new communist government was greatly concerned with social rather than individual needs and by assuming responsibility for all health care of chinese citizens and enlisting citizen participation, Mao greatly enlarged the total health care system including psychiatry (Chesneaux 1979). Disease prevention was emphasized, and both modern and traditional psychiatrists were included in the effort. By 1957 there were almost three times more psychiatric beds and eight times the number of chinese psychiatric doctors than there had been at the time of the Bowman Report in 1947.

In 1958 China's increased efforts at modernization in Mao's "Great Leap Forward" were felt in psychiatry. Outpatient treatment was expanded; child guidance clinics were opened and psychologists were added to the mental health team (Taipale 1973). China's great concern with the problems of schizophrenia, and neurasthenia, a mixture of neurotic psychosomatic symptoms, led to increased epidemiological study. Mental health workers interviewed two million people in the 50's and analyzed data alleged to demonstrate that schizophrenia had a morbidity of only .98% to 1% per thousand, one tenth as high as in the capitalistic West. It has, however, been speculated that underreporting by western standards and relegation of many cases to political and ideological categories may have removed them from psychiatric purview.

Soviet Influences

Soon after the emergence of Mao's People's Republic of China, and with the rejection of western psychiatric theories, the impact of soviet psychiatric thought became felt in chinese psychiatric theory and practice. Soviet texts were used in the teaching of psychiatry, and the neurological theories of the great russian psychologist, Ivan Pavlov, emphasizing biological aspects of mental illness, replaced western ideas of unconscious personality conflicts.

Traditional chinese ideas blended well with russian influence. Pavlov's ideas of inhibition of cortical brain regions and their relationship to specific cutaneous areas were compatible with chinese theories of acupuncture. Soviet ideas emphasizing the value of work, social consciousness, willpower, environment, and reeducation, found much support in the new chinese republic, whose ancient traditions had always stressed proper moral choice, group responsibility and education.

The political writings of Chairman Mao were studied by psychiatric staff and patients alike, and were used in treatment situations to organize thinking along proper lines and to thus promote correct understanding. Gradually as soviet chinese friendship declined, soviet psychiatric influence waned and the role of Mao's writings as a therapeutic instrument gained greater prominence. China had begun to develop her own individual psychiatric method and direction with the writings of Chairman Mao.

The Cultural Revolution and Its Effects 1965–1969

From 1965–1969 China underwent great social upheaval as loyal maoist, "Red Guards" swept through the country in an effort to eliminate political revisionism and to unite all levels of society under a purified maoist ideology by vigorous reassessment and reeducation. Psychiatric research and training were disrupted and hospitals reorganized under a treatment team approach. Staff and patients were encouraged to become more politically minded in all aspects of life and in psychiatric situations. Political elements were introduced into the management of hospitals. More psychiatric education and training was offered lower staff members whose responsibilities increased, and traditional medicine received official recognition in psychiatric treatment.

With end of the cultural revolution more medical schools emerged. The use of western antipsychotic drugs (phenothiazines, and lithium salts) was combined with traditional methods such acupuncture for hallucinations, mania or stupor with an alleged remission rate of 60% to 70%. Electricity was applied to acupuncture needles for daily stimulation over month long periods (Taipale and Taipale 1973).

The aftermath of the Cultural Revolution appears to have been the broadening of staff education, and the increased use of a team approach among psychiatric personel. There was as well, increased rapprochment of western and traditional chinese psychiatric treatments in various combinations. Increased emphasis was placed upon the social causes of mental illness which was understood to arise from overconcern with personal interests as opposed to the collective social goals espoused in Mao's writings.

The New Mental Health Care Delivery System in People's Republic in China

Following the Cultural Revolution, revisions in the chinese health care system greatly expanded rural health care, and created an organized referral system starting from the local part time para-medical "barefoot" doctor working in production brigades with fellow workers.

The referral process in rural China is initiated by a "barefoot" doctor at the brigade level consisting of approximately 10 villages for which there is a brigade clinic. From this clinic a patient may be sent to a larger commune (16,000 people) hospital, to a county (50,000 people) hospital, or to a district hospital. A district, consisting of 4 million people is the "secondary" more specialized level of care. The highest level of medical sophistication and specialization, "tertiary" care is that of the municipal or provincial hospital, usually located in urban centers, often associated with medical colleges and having specialized subunits.

Urban referrals begin at workplace or neighborhood clinics at the primary level, rising to neighborhood or urban district hospitals at the secondary level and then to tertiary centers. While psychiatric cases may follow the above routes, family, local groups or commune staff may petition psychiatric problems directly to tertiary centers for treatment.

Contrary to popular belief, health care in China is not fully state supported. Payment for medical and psychiatric care is by health insurance which varies according to occupation. Certain labor and party organizers receive complete insurance coverage, while peasants and workers on smaller collectives receive only partial coverage, occasionally bearing substantial cost burdens themselves (Henderson 1982:). This no doubt increases the appeal of traditional, less expensive, treatment methods among those with less insurance coverage.

Hospital Care

Consideration of the issues of hospital care and research is best attempted by a look at China's tertiary care psychiatric facilities representing the current state of the art in psychiatric care. Such an example, The Shanghai Psychiatric Hospital Number Two was built in 1958 as a 1000 bed institution served by a staff of 556 people with 15 administrators, all of whom are psychiatrists themselves, some with training in traditional medicine as well.

This hospital, representing the best of psychiatric care stresses the widely favored community approach to hospital treatment. This involves structured group activities for all patients, most of whom carry a diagnosis of schizophrenia. Few individual rooms exist in order to discourage withdrawal and isolation. The hospital boasts game rooms, T.V. and occupational therapy. The staff to patient ratio is one to one, with one psychiatrist per dozen patients. Average patient age is 30, and average length of stay is 3 months with discharge to home or outpatient care as needed.

Presentation of cases to visitors in 1982 (Collins 1982) by clinical psychologists and psychiatrists appeared similar to the western hospital model with group and limited "suason" therapy consisting of discussion. Psychiatrists appeared quite familiar with major western neuroleptic drugs which were replacing electroshock therapy for depression as well as replacing the traditional herbs and acupuncture more common a decade earlier (Ratnavale 1973:1084). Acupuncture and herbal methods appear to be more prominently in use at lower levels of the medical hierarchy, and in rural outpatient settings. At the tertiary level trends appear to favor western methods especially in inpatient settings.

Research in Mental Illness

Teaching hospitals such as the Shanghai Psychiatric Hospital described above, and the Peking Institute of Mental Health conduct much of the psychiatric research in China. In China mental illness is seen largely as a biological phenomenon, an idea compatible with both chinese medical tradition, and with some sectors of western psychiatric theory. In addition the great chinese interest in schizophrenia, a major mental illness with rather clear biological predispositions, also encourages a biological rather than a psychological focus.

Consequently chinese psychiatric research falls into four general areas, that of biochemistry, of genetics, of neurophysiology, and of psychiatric epidemiology. Studies of schizophrenia often attempt to clarify the roles and the effects of traditional remedies upon various symptom complexes. An interesting combination of the old and the new is the recent use of computers employed in classification and prescription of ancient herbal remedies for mental and physical illness.

This biological orientation reveals itself in chinese medical education which regards psychiatry merely as an aspect of general medicine. Consequently, Chinese medical schools, unlike their U.S. counterparts, do not offer their medical students courses in psychiatry but only about 20 hours of interviewing techniques instead. (Nutter 1983).

The Psychological Dilemma: Outpatient Treatment

As has been described, most psychiatric inpatients in China carry a diagnosis of schizophrenia which is thought of as neurobiological in origin and treated with drugs, hospital structure, and occasionally by traditional methods. Less severe psychiatric illness considered to be neurotic and of psychological origin in the West are considered in China to be problems in the area of education or social maladjustment. Such a view is reflected in the chinese diagnostic category of "sexual nonconformity" unknown in the West (Wilson 1983).

Thus chinese psychiatry is confronted with a conceptual disharmony. Having rejected western psychological theories of unconscious neurotic causation, and having leaned heavily upon biological explanations and chemical treatments for the major psychotic illnesses, the Chinese are left without a clear theoretical basis for diagnosis and treatment of the many non psychotic conditions that comprise their psychiatric outpatient population. This population is of substantial size. The outpatient population of the Shanghai Psychiatric Hospital comprises 400 patients daily, mostly suffering neurotic and psychosomatic conditions. Despite this fact the diagnoses of depression, phobias, obsessions or hysteria so commonly employed in the West are rarely used at all. Neurasthenia, other psychosomatic categories and stress reactions are however often used as diagnostic categories.

The rarity of depression, so commonly diagnosed outside of China, is assumed by chinese psychiatrists to be due to its appearance in chinese medical clinics where it manifests itself in terms of physical symptoms rather than by the less socially acceptable complaints of unhappiness and pessimism. Peking and Hwangchao psychiatrists explained that they did not see cases of sexual neuroses, homosexuality, alocholism, drug abuse, or suicide although they understood them to be common in overseas chinese communities (Kleinman, Mechanic 1979). Unpublished reports of foreign psychiatric contacts with private chinese citizens however, suggest that when such problems as these arise in less than extreme form, they are often hidden to avoid negative social consequences thereby escaping medical notice.

Outpatient treatment of discharged hospital schizophrenics generally continues the format of their hospital treatment. They receive their former medication. They are prepared for reentry into the community by group discussions, and they are returned, if possible to former employment with the assistance and intervention of hospital personel. Patients too sick for such placement are treated in a health center or clinic with therapy groups that provide work, recreation and medicine (Wilson, Hutchinson 1983).

Less is known about treatment of the non psychotic outpatient in China. Bermann in 1968 and Ratnavale in 1973 observed that combinations of western and traditional medicines, acupuncture, and group discussions have been offered on an outpatient basis. They described, at that time, group therapy outpatient sessions consisting of the reading and discussions of Chairman Mao's writings to correct "false ideas", to encourage social responsibility and to formulate a recovery plan. It is likely that since the death of Mao and the lessening of his influence the direct use of his writings in therapy may have declined somewhat or even passed into disuse entirely but this is not yet known. Most likely is the uneven or intermittent use of his writings to illustrate principles of social rehabilitation in different therapy groups as may seem judicious from time to time. Such changes were seen in a 1985 CBS television special on China. Shown were the efforts of a citizen counselor exhorting a father to become more considerate of his wife, and more accepting of the sex of their newly born daughter. Another episode dealt with the kleptomania of a young woman who was lectured severly by court and counselors for her lack of social responsibility and who ultimately repented her deviation from socialist principles becoming happily rehabilitated.

It seems that personal problems when not viewed as mental illness are thought of in a community or socialist context. This is particularly so when mental symptoms take the form of behavior rather than psychosomatic or affective expression. Thus chinese non biological approaches to mental problems which in the West would be considered personal in origin, requiring individual study, rely in China upon the power of political and social reeducation, usually in group situations. Culture, work family and community life are often enlisted to promote recovery from mental illness or personal problems although no theory of how such interventions effect recovery has yet been devised by the Chinese. Nonetheless such methods appear to rely heavily upon reinforcing traditional moral attitudes regarding group responsibility harmony and affiliation. Group awareness in China and its applications may differ from our own, yet prove instructive for both East and West to understand.

Most recently chinese psychiatrists have shown a growing interest in western diagnostic categories, especially of the neuroses (Michels 1984). Whether or not this represents a possible expansion of chinese thinking about mental illness, or a blurring of former diagnostic boundaries cannot yet be determined, but should prove interesting to observe as chinese exposure to western psychiatric knowledge increases.

Treatment of Children and the Elderly

In keeping with concepts of group participation and harmony concepts of chinese mental hygiene, concentrate upon
the proper rearing of children and the proper role and treatment of the aged. Each is a population vulnerable to mental
illness and heavily dependent upon social attitudes (Sidel
1972). Owing to high percentage of working mothers most
children are raised in state nurseries where professional care-
takers feed, train, and later educate them to social responsibility. The Chinese feel that such upbringing eliminates
juvenile delinquency as known in the West (Lazure 1964).
However even today, little is known about the nature and
prevailance of juvenile delinquency in China which appears to
treat social deviance more repressively than the West. The
direct medical treatment of the mental disorders of childhood,
called child psychiatry is quite limited in China having fallen
into disfavor during the Cultural Revolution. It is only now
beginning to emerge as a speciality of its own.

The aged infirm, for the most part still cared for by their
family, are provided with financial and medical support and
with workers' residences if necessary (Chesneaux 1970). Attempts are made to keep the elderly, even those with mental
infirmity, productive within the mainstream of society as
much as possible. The usual spectrum of mental disorders
such as the organic dementias, psychoses and geriatric de-
pressions are recognized in the chinese geriatric population,
and are usually treated in mental health centers. Mental
health centers for the elderly offer work, both western traditional medicines, exercise, and recreation to aged mentally ill.
Geriatric therapy groups have been reported to produce high
levels of recovery from mental illness as a result of discussion,
diet, and an unvarying work schedule (Wilson and Hutchinson 1983).

Conclusions

China is a country with a distinguished system of medicine
reaching back 3000 years in which mental illness has never

been separated from its somatic aspects (Yates 1979). Traditional chinese treatments of diet, rest, acupuncture, herbalism and environmental adjustments preceed recorded history.

The Chinese Peoples' Republic, following a period of soviet influence in medicine, and then a heavily ideological maoist period of cultural revolution, is now attempting to employ western biological technology in psychiatric illness while preserving its traditional methods. Psychiatric research is largely biochemical, but inpatient treatments, and more especially outpatient treatments are psychological, group oriented, and moralistic within a framework of traditional chinese social values.

Traditional medical and psychiatric treatments are still widely employed among the rural chinese population and the lower social classes where they are found to be both acceptable and cost effective. In addition traditional medical approaches are taught in both general medical schools and in special traditional medical schools. In their search for effective psychiatric treatment methods, the Chinese have attempted to combine traditional and modern approaches. These approaches coexist in varying pragmatic combinations as China continues to attempt her own unique synthesis of traditional and modern psychiatric care for the benefit of her people.

Bibliography

Bermann, Gregorio (1968) "Mental Health in China" pp. 223–261 in Ari Kiev (ed.) Psychiatry in the Communist World. N.Y. Science House

Chang, Margaret (1983) "Nursing in China, Three Perspectives" American Journal of Nursing March 1983: 389–391

Chesneaux, Jean (1979) China The People's Republic 1949–1976 English Translation of La Chine (Pantheon Asia Library) N.Y. Random House Inc.

Collins, James (1982) "Psychiatry in China" Journal of the National Medical Assoc. vol. 74 no. 10 993–998

Haldipur, C.V. (1980) "The Idea of 'Cultural' Psychiatry: A Comment on the Foundations of Cultural Psychiatry" Comprehensive Psychiatry: vol 21, no. 3 206–211

Henderson, Gail E., and Myron S. Cohen (1982) "Health Care in the People's Republic of China: A View From Inside the System." American Journal of Public Health vol. 72 no. 11: 1238–1245

Kleinman, Arthur, and David Mechanic (1979) "Some Observations of Mental Illness and Its Treatment in The People's Republic of China." Journal of Nervous and Mental Disease vol.167 No.5: 267–274

Koran, Lorrin (1972) "Psychiatry in Mainland China History and Recent Status." American Journal of Psychiatry vol.128 No.8:970–977

Li, Dun J. (1971) The Ageless Chinese. 2nd edition N.Y. Scribners

Liu, Xiehe (1981) "Psychiatry in Traditional Chinese Medicine." British Journal of Psychiatry vol.138: 429–433

Mechanic, David (1984) "Chinese Have Made Strides in Health System." American Medical News Jan. 27, 1984 p. 26

Michels, Robert (1984) "A Debate on DSM III, First Rebuttal." American Journal of Psychiatry vol.141 No.4: p.549

Nutter, Donald (1983) "Medical Education In The People's Republic of China." Journal of Medical Education vol 58:555–561

Ratnavale, David (1973) "Psychiatry in Shanghai China: Observations in 1973." American Journal of Psychiatry Vol.130 No.10: 1082–1087

Sidel, Ruth (1972) Women and Child Care in the People's Republic of China N.Y. Hill and Wang

Sidel, Victor (1982) "Medical Care in China: Equity vs. Modernization." American Journal of Public Health vol.172 No.11:1224–1226

Taipale, Vappu and Likka Taipale (1973) "Chinese Psychiatry, A Visit to a Chinese Mental Hospital" Archives of General Psychiatry Vol.29: 313–316

Tseng, Wen-Shing (1973) "The Development of Psychiatric Concepts in Traditional Medicine." Archives of General Psychiatry Vol.29:569–575

Yates, Robin (1979) "The History of China." Diversion Magazine pub. Diversion Publications N.Y. Vol.7 No.2 (February) pp. 25–27 and pp.42–44

Wilson, Holly and Sally Hutchinson (1983) "Psychiatric Diagnosis Range From Depression and Violence to Social and Sexual Nonconformity." American Journal of Nursing March 1983: 393–395

CHAPTER 3

Industrialization and Health Care in Taiwan

Wen-Hui Tsai

Examined are the improvements and probems in health-care service in Taiwan during a period of rapid industrialization and economic growth from the 1959's to the 1980's. The problems addressed in particular are the lack of drug regulation and the conflict between traditional Chinese medicine and western trained physicians.

I. Industrialization and Socio-Economic Development

TAIWAN'S ECONOMIC DEVELOPMENT FOR THE PAST THIRTY years has been exceptional. Economist Herman Kahn (1979) in his discussion of world economic development singled out Taiwan, along with South Korea and Japan, as "heroes" of development, nations which have lifted themselves from abject poverty to middle-income levels in less than a decade and are now within a decade or so of becoming fully mature industrial economies. John C. H. Fei *et al* (1979) and Walter Galenson (1979) have also called Taiwan's success a "miracle," while Richard E. Barrett and Martin King Whyte (1982) have

35

labelled Taiwan a "deviant case" of the dependency theory of development.

Industrialization and economic growth in Taiwan are not an overnight success story. Rather they have been achieved through careful planning and effective implementation of plans. From 1953 to 1981, six long-range economic plans were launched and effectively implemented. As a result, the national economy has shifted from agriculture-oriented to industrial-oriented, from import-oriented to export-oriented, and from relative poverty to prosperity.

As clearly demonstrated in Table 1, the non-agricultural population in Taiwan steadily increased between 1951 and 1979, with almost 70 percent of the total population engaged in non-agricultural activities. Such a shift of a large proportion of population from agricultural activities to industrial activities has increased the relative importance of industrial products in the net domestic product. As Table 1 shows, industrial products occupied 13.1% of the net domestic product in 1951, and were increased to 34.32% in 1979. Volumes of gross national product during the same period increased from US$2,110.5 millions to US$24,751.6 millions; per-capita income increased from US$246 to US$1,228; and the over-all national economy grew at a very impressive rate during the period. When the Nationalist government of Chiang Kai-shek moved to Taiwan in 1949, Taiwan was predominantly an agricultural society, with a large proportion of its population residing in rural areas. The economic boom of the past thirty years, especially in the 1960's and 1970's, not only increased the nation's wealth dramatically, but also changed the social structure of Taiwan.

One of the major changes in Taiwan during the period was rapid urbanization. As new technology and industry located in or close to urban centers, population started to move from rural to urban areas. In Taiwan, we see the rapid increase of urban population: In 1951 about 51% of the population on the island lived in urban areas, but by 1979 it had increased to 67.1% (Tsai, 1982). Moreover, the evidence also shows that this urban population was concentrated in a few large metropolitan areas. For example, in 1957 only 27.5% of the island's population lived in urban areas with a population of 100,000 or more, but by 1978 the percentage had increased to 45.5%. At the same time, the number of urban areas with a population of 100,000 or more also increased, from 8 in 1957 to 17 in 1978. In other words, almost half of Taiwan's population was living in 17 large urban cities by 1978. Government reports (Executive Yuan, 1979; Ministry of Interior Affairs, (1982) further show that almost half of Taiwan's urban population is concentrated in four major metropolises with a population of 500,000 or more. Other changes are also evident. As we can see from Table 1, the overall quality of life for the people in Taiwan has been improved characterized by a steady decline of the unemployment rate, a better distribution of family income, the lowering of the illiteracy rate, and an increase of leisure.

11. Improvements in Health Care: A Statistical Portrait

Health Conditions vary greatly from society to society and within societies, but most scholars seem to be in agreement that health conditions throughout the developing world are substantially inferior to those in industrialized societies. Researchers have found that industrialization and the subsequent economic and social development bring improvements in the general health of a population, and that the more a society is industrialized, the more developed its medical and health-care system become (World Bank, 1980; Navarro, 1979). During the past thirty years, economic growth and social development have been accompanied by improving health care.

Health and Medical-Care Facilities. The number of public and private hospitals and clinics has steadily increased. The data for the period between 1961 and 1980 on public hospitals and clinics operated by central and local governments reflect a slow but steady increase. In 1961 there were 1,089 public hospitals and clinics and they were increased to 1,295 in 1980.

Table 1
Selected Indicators of Taiwan's Overall Quality of Life, 1951–1979

Indicator	1951	1956	1961	1966	1971	1976	1979
% of non-agricultural population in total population	47.13	49.96	50.96	55.31	60.26	66.30	67.74
% of industrial product in net domestic product	13.01	14.53	16.99	20.34	28.90	32.55	34.32
Gross national product (Million US$)	2110.5	3230.2	4525.5	7255.0	11979.6	18318.4	24751.6
Per capita income (US$)	246	316	371	520	770	1039	1288
Economic growth rate (%)	NA	5.50	6.83	9.01	12.90	13.48	8.08
Unemployment rate (%)	4.4	3.6	4.1	3.0	1.7	2.0	1.3
% urban population in total population	51.0	52.8	53.3	56.7	60.4	66.3	67.1
Income share of bottom 20% of all households	NA	NA	7.5	7.9	8.4	8.9	8.6
Illiteracy Rate (%)	43.4	37.1	25.9	23.1	14.0	12.1	10.7
Number of leisure hours per month	NA	NA	NA	492	503	509	508

(Sources: *National Income of the Republic of China*, 1979. *Statistical Yearbook of the Republic of China*, 1979. *Graphical Survey of the Economy of Taiwan*, the Republic of China, 1980.)

Similarly, the number of private hospitals and clinics experienced a rapid increase in the 1970's, from 6,338 units in 1971 to 9,993 in 1980. A comparison between public and private hospitals and clinics during the 1970's thus indicates a faster growth in the private sector. Taking 1971 as the base year for comparison, the index for public hospitals and clinics in 1980 was 108, while the index for private hospitals and clinics in 1980 was 157.7).

The growth of health and medical-care facilities can also be found in the increase of hospital beds. The number of hospital beds per 10,000 population has increased from 3.70 in 1961 to 22.41 in 1980. The expansion of hospital beds is attributable to the growth in the private sector of health and medical facilities, as discussed earlier.

Medical and Para-Medical Personnel Structure. The total number of medical and para-medical personnel during the past 20 years increased from 12,678 in 1961 to 66,278 in 1985, a net increase of 53,600.

A detailed analysis of the medical and para-medical personnel growth reveals the increase occurred largely among specialists other than physicians and dentists. As shown in Table 2, although physicians constituted more than half of the medical professionals in the early 1960's, they have steadily declined as a percentage of the medical pool ever since. In 1985, physicians accounted for only 25.6% of the total medical and para-medical personnel, which reflected a decline of 26.3% during the past 25 years. The percentage of dentists experienced a similar decline, from 6.3% in 1961 to 5.2% in 1985. Nurses and pharmacists, however, have both enjoyed a significant increase. In 1961, nurses constituted 12.5% and pharmacists 7.5% of the total medical and para-medical professionals, but the percentages in 1985 showed 36.6% for nurses and 24.6% for pharmacists. The expansion within the medical and para-medical professions in Taiwan has been largely in the two specialists of nursing and pharmacists.

This trend is due to the fact that government imposes extremely tight regulations on the licensing of both physicians

and dentists, but not on nurses and pharmacists. Also the
medical education of physicians and dentists is offered at
college and post-college levels, while nursing and pharmacy
programs can be offered in junior colleges and vocational high
school.

Health Conditions of the General Population. The steady
expansions of both health and medical care facilities and staffs
have provided better health care for the general population of
Taiwan. The number of physicians per 10,000 population increased from 6.0 in 1961 to 7.6 in 1980, dentists from 0.7 to
1.2, pharmacists from 0.9 to 6.8, and nurses from 1.5 to 6.6.
At the same time, the number of hospital beds per 10,000
population also increased, from 3.70 in 1961 to 22.4 in 1980.

Household expenditures for medical and health care have
also shown a steady increase, both in real-dollar amount and
in proportion of the family total budget. In 1961, the amount
spent for medical and health care per household was
US$25.00 and about 4.2% of the household budget; in 1980,
the amount was increased to US$300,000 and 5.5% of the
household budget.

With a rapidly growing national economy, the government
in Taiwan has invested more and more capital in the improve-

Table 2
Medical and Para-Medical Personnel Structure

Year	Total	%	Physicians	Dentists	Nurses	Pharmacists	Others
1961	12,678	100	51.9	6.3	12.5	7.5	21.8
1964	13,282	100	50.0	6.1	13.9	8.4	21.6
1967	15,820	100	49.0	5.1	15.4	9.6	20.9
1970	18,992	100	39.6	4.3	19.2	12.1	24.8
1973	20,447	100	40.9	4.9	20.2	17.7	16.3
1976	32,008	100	35.5	4.3	26.7	17.1	16.4
1979	39,614	100	33.7	4.5	28.4	17.1	16.8
1982	49,899	100	28.8	5.2	30.2	28.2	7.6
1985	66,278	100	25.6	5.2	36.6	24.6	8.0

(Sources: *Statistical Yearbook of the Republic of China, 1981.* Taipei: Executive
Yuan, Table 222, pp. 632–633. *Social Indicators of the Republic of China, 1985.*
Taipei: Executive Yuan, Table 67, pp. 226–227.)

ment of health and medical care. Statistics show that in 1961 government health-related expenditures total US$1,076,877.2, a figure increased to US$196,778,000 in 1982 (National Health Administration, 1982:30).

As a result of the expansion of medical and health-care services, the health conditions of the general population in Taiwan have been improved over the years. One indicator of such an improvement is the decline of mortality rates. During the period between 1961 and 1985, as shown in Table 3, the crude death rates declined from 6.6 per 1,000 population to 4.8 per 1,000 population; the mortality rates for newborn children declined from 32.7 to 7.4; and the maternal mortality rates from 9.6 to 1.0. Meanwhile, the average life expectancy has been extended from 62.3 years for men and 67.7 for women to 70.8 years for men and 75.8 years for women.

In summary, increased in national wealth and personal income have contributed to an expansion of medical and health-care service which, in turn, has provided better health and a longer life expectancy for the population in Taiwan.

III. Old and Newly Emerging Problems

There is no doubt that medical and health care in Taiwan has been greatly improved during the recent period of a rapid socio-economic growth; people are in general healthier and live longer. Nevertheless, some old problems persist, and some new ones have arisen.

Probably the most troublesome issue facing a developing nation like Taiwan is the absence of regulation of medical service and practice. The World Bank's 1980 report on health problems in improving health do not result from the complexity of medical technology, and only partially from the scarcity of financial resources; rather, "they derive principally from problems in the design and implementation of policy, management, and logistics" (1980:7). In Taiwan, there is no regulatory agency to oversee medical services and practice. When a mishap occurs, it is not the fault of any medical

Table 3
Crude Death Rates, Mortality Rates for Newborn Children, Maternal Mortality Rates, and Average Life Expectancy

Year	Crude Death Rates	Mortality Rates for Newborn Children (per 1,000 live births)	Maternal Mortality Rates (per 10,000 live births)	Average Life Expectancy	
				Men	Women
1961	6.6	32.7	9.6	62.3	67.7
1964	5.6	25.5	7.9	63.8	69.2
1967	5.4	21.1	6.2	64.2	69.7
1970	4.9	17.4	4.0	66.1	71.1
1973	4.8	16.2	4.0	67.7	72.8
1976	4.7	12.9	3.0	68.8	73.7
1979	4.7	11.0	1.7	69.4	74.5
1982	4.7	8.9	1.9	70.2	75.1
1985	4.8	7.4	1.0	70.8	75.8

(Source: *Social Indicators of the Republic of China, 1985*. Taipei: Executive Yuan. Table 68 & 69, pp. 229–233.)

personnel, but the misfortune of the patient. Abuse of prescribed drugs is wide-spread. Not only does the government fail to establish guidelines for the use of these drugs, but also people are allowed to buy any drug they want at drugstores, with or without a physician's prescription. The problem is complicated by the fact that many drug manufacturers from industrialized nations such as the United States, Germany, and Japan have used Taiwan as a test site for their newly developed, untested drugs and for dumping unsafe drugs which failed to receive approval from government agencies in their home countries (China Times Weekly, 1983; Silverman, 1982). A few incidents have been reported in recent years in Taiwan (Kao, 1983).

Another problem in recent years is a growing conflict between traditional Chinese medical practitioners and Western-trained medical professionals. Industrialization and its subsequent socio-economic effects in Taiwan have turned people away from many things traditional, for they are labelled "backward." Traditional Chinese medicine is one of these areas. Of the 30 medical schools in Taiwan today, none provides training in traditional Chinese medicine. Data in Table 4 shows that although the number of doctors of Chinese traditional medicine grew from 1,674 to 1,758 between 1961 and 1982, the number of Western trained physicians grew much faster, from 4,900 to 12,594, during the same period. Moreover, traditional medicine is offered only in small, private clinics; the large government-operated public hospitals and clinics do not offer any traditional Chinese medicines, nor do they use traditional practices, except sometimes acupuncture.

Still another problem for the health and medical profession in Taiwan is the emergence of new diseases caused by industrial pollution. Industrialization in Taiwan has been achieved so rapidly that there was no time for industrialists or government officials to pay attention to air and water pollution caused by industrial-waste dumping. In recent years, food contamination and poisoning, industrial accidents, and deaths caused by pollution have all been on the rise. Taiwan's small size and dense population make the situation ever worse.

Table 4
Modern Western Trained Physicians and Doctors of Chinese Medicine

Year	Number of Modern Western Trained Physicians	Number of Doctors of Chinese Medicine
1961	4,900	1,674
1964	4,983	1,666
1967	5,320	1,587
1970	5,092	1,384
1973	6,817	1,550
1976	9,926	1,435
1979	11,554	1,615
1982	12,594	1,758

(Source: *Health Statistics: Republic of China, 1982*. Taipei: National Health Administration. Table 29, pp. 84–85.)

Table 5 shows the ten leading causes of death between 1961 and 1985. It is evident that death caused by cerebrovascular diseases, malignant neoplasms, accidents, hypertensive diseases, and cirrhosis of the liver have been increasing, while death caused by pneumonia, bronchitis, emphysema and asthma, tuberculosis, and suicide declined.

Finally, something must be said about the uneven distribution of physicians in Taiwan. A recent study (Chang, 1983) found that 49% of physicians and 21% of hospitals are concentrated in Taipei City alone, even though the city's population has only 13% of the island's total population. Another 5% of physicians are in the second-largest city, Kaohsuing which has 6% of the total population. In other words, more than half of the physicians and large proportion of the hospitals are located in the two largest cities in Taiwan. Another study (Land, 1983) discovered that the number of physicians in the two largest cities is one per 750 population; in cities with population over 100,000, the ratio is one physician per 900; in cities with population over 50,000, the ratio is one physician per 1,300 population; in cities with population of 10,000, the ratio is one physician per 1,900; and in rural counties, the ratio is one physicians per 3,869. It is clear, then, that higher degrees of urbanization bring increased availability of physicians in Taiwan today. A related problem is the fact that about 25% of medical-college graduates and 40% of pharmacists now reside abroad, with a great majority in the United States.

V. Concluding Remarks

During the past 20 years, Taiwan has enjoyed one of the most successful socio-economic growth rates found in developing nations. Taiwan's expanded economy, better income distribution, and other social developments have made improvements in health and medical care possible. The years have brought health and medical care facilities, medical and para-medical personnel, and improved health conditions. Nevertheless, a few problems have emerged such as the lack

Table 5
Death Rates by the Ten Leading Causes
in Per 100,000 Persons

Year	Cerebro-Vascular Diseases	Malignant Neoplasma	Accidents	Heart Disease	Pneumonia	Hypertensive Disease	Cirrhosis of Liver	Bronchitis Emphysema and Asthma	Tuberculosis	Suicide and Self-Inflicted Injuries
1961	49.86	41.73	38.90	44.00	65.88	11.48	10.88	15.61	42.13	16.36
1964	63.77	46.84	37.50	35.13	46.42	9.09	12.52	25.94	39.71	18.74
1967	67.70	51.40	41.45	37.15	38.52	8.80	12.31	20.11	35.64	13.50
1970	66.22	55.52	45.12	36.41	30.84	8.40	13.23	14.36	28.38	12.41
1973	73.39	61.89	50.04	40.68	28.99	13.17	16.11	18.28	24.72	10.20
1976	74.40	64.04	53.46	43.46	24.45	14.40	16.45	14.88	19.32	8.75
1979	75.51	70.58	64.40	40.64	18.81	17.86	17.03	15.44	15.42	9.91
1982	77.99	78.66	60.37	43.82	12.31	17.61	16.95	14.92	13.00	12.30
1985	76.42	85.02	58.97	43.52	—*	18.08	16.48	13.98	—*	11.92

Note: Both Pneumonia and Tuberculosis were no longer among the ten leading causes of death in Taiwan in 1985.

(Source: *Social Indicators of the Republic of China, 1985,* Taipei: Executive Yuan. Table 69, pp. 232–233.)

of drug regulation, the conflict between traditional Chinese medicine and Western-trained physicians, pollution-related diseases, and the great concentration of physicians in urban areas. All these problems are not serious yet, but they do need attention from the government and the public so that they can be contained and resolved.

References

Brenner, M. Harvey (1980) "Industrialization and Economic Growth: Estimates of their Effects on the Health of Populations." Pp.65–115 in M. Harvey Brenner, A. Mooney, and T. J. Nagy, eds., Assessing the Contributions of the Social Sciences to Health. AAAS Selected Symposium 26. Boulder, Col.: Westview.

Bryant, John (1969) Health and the Developing World. Ithaca: Cornell.

Cahill, Kevin M. ed. (1976) Health and Development. N.Y.: Orbis Books.

Chang, Ly-yun (1983) "A Preliminary Report on the Study of Health Manpower Distribution in Taiwan." Chinese Journal of Sociology. 7:133–156.

China Times Weekly (1983) "Taiwan's Environment Problems." China Times Weekley. 235:15–18.

Executive Yuan, The. (1979a) National Income of the Republic of China. Taipei: Executive Yuan. (1979) Statistical Yearbook of the Republic of China. Taipei: Executive Yuan. (1980) Graphical Survey of the Republic of China. Taipei: Executive Yuan. (1982a) Social Welfare Indicators of the Republic of China. Taipei: Executive Yuan. (1982b) Statistical Yearbook of the Republic of China. Taipei: Executive Yuan. (1982c) Social Indicators of the Republic of China. Taipei: Executive Yuan. (1985) Social Indicators of the Republic of China. Taipei: Executive Yuan.

Fei, John C.H., Gustav Ranis, and Shirley W.Y. Kuo (1979) Growth with Equity: The Taiwan Case. New York: Oxford.

Galenson, Walter, ed. Economic Growth and Structural Change in Taiwan. Ithaca: Cornell. (1979)

Grosse, R. N. and O. Harkavy (1980) "The Role of Health in Development." Social Sciences and Medicine. 140:165–69.

Kahn, Herman (1979) World Economic Development, 1979 and Beyond. Boulder, Col: Westview.

Kao, Shi-ching (1983) The Concern Over the Quality of Life. Taipei: Center for the Study of Quality of Life.

Kleinman, A., ed. (1975) Medicine in Chinese Cultures: Comparative Studies of Health Care in Chines and Other Societies. Bethesda, Maryland: Fogarty International Center, National Institute of Health.

Lang, Chung-fu (1983) The Distribution of Medical Doctors in Taiwan. An unpublished Report.

National Health Administration (1982) Health Statistics, Republic of China, 1982. Taipei: National Health Administration.

Navarro, Vincente (1982) "Radicalism, Marxism, and Medicine." International Journal of Health Service. (13.2): 179–202.

Silverman, Milton, Philip R. Lee, and Mia Lydecker (1982) "The Drugging of the Third World." International Journal of Health Service (12:4): 585–96.

Tsai, Wen-hui (1982) "Industrialization and Urbanization in Taiwan" Journal of Sociology, 15:63–81.

Weatherby, Norman L., Charles B. Nam, and Larry W. Tsaac (1983) "Developmeng, Inequality, Health Care, and Mortality at the Older Ages: A Cross-National Analysis." Demography (20:1):27–41.

World Bank (1980) Health. New York: The World Bank.

CHAPTER 4

Childbearing and the Training of Traditional Birth Attendants in Haiti

Suzanne Allman

Discussed are current practices of child birth in Haiti. Based on in-depth interviews with mothers and traditional birth attendants, this research looks at a program to improve childbirth practices through the training of indigenous midwives, who assist over 70 percent of the women who deliver in Haiti. This program appears to have stimulated poor, rural women to seek pre-natal care. Through the immunization with tetanus toxoid of pregnant women, there is a reduction in neo-natal tetanus, a major cause of infant death in Haiti. The low cost of this program, and its enthusiastic acceptance by both mothers and midwives, suggests an openness to such primary health care interventions through integration of modern and traditional practitioners.

Introduction

OVER TWO THIRDS OF THE WORLD'S INFANTS ARE CURrently born at home, attended by indigenous midwives. These traditional birth attendants, (further on referred to as TBA's) assist the majority of mothers in confronting childbearing in environments characterized by poor sanitation, high levels of infection and disease, far from the highly organized, sophisticated health care people in the developed world take for granted (Simpson-Hebert et al., 1980). This is the case in Haiti, where in 1983 less than 30 percent of women delivered in hospitals or other health facilities. Although lack of resources in Haiti precludes a dramatic change in childbearing practices, which would lead to high percentages of hospital compared to home deliveries, efforts by the Haitian Division of Family Hygiene (DHF) over the last ten years, based on previous studies and projects to train TBAs in better methods of delivery, have lead to some important improvements in the conditions that mothers and their infants now face.

Background

Haiti, a Caribbean country with a population of over 5 million according to the 1982 Census, shares the Western one-third of the island of Hispaniola with the Dominican Republic. The country is the poorest in Latin America (per capita GNP is estimated at below US $300 in 1984). Most of the Haitian population (over 70 percent) still live in rural areas and earn a meager livelihood from agriculture.

Although major efforts have been made since the late 1970's to improve basic health care, conditions are still very bad. Infant mortality is estimated at between 124–150 deaths per 1000 births, child and adult mortality are high, and life expectancy at birth is around 50 years. Diarrhea, infectious diseases and malnutrition are major causes of death especially among the young. The crude birth rate is estimated at 36 per 1000 for the 1980–1984 period and less than 5 percent of women at risk were using modern contraceptives according to the 1983 Contraceptive Prevalence Survey (Allman, James, 1982).

Giving Birth in Haiti

Between 1980 and 1982 the author interviewed and tape recorded 20 women concerning their experiences in giving birth. Interviews generally lasted between 1 and 2 hours and were conducted in Haitian creole. These qualitative data provide the major source of information on current childbirth practices in Haiti, and are reported in detail elsewhere (Allman, Susan, 1983).

In rural areas of Haiti most deliveries take place at home in a one-room poorly furnished, dirt-floored thatched hut with no sanitary facilities and little furniture. Some babies are delivered in the field, while their mothers are at market, or while the mother is collecting water or doing other errands. The mother usually delivers in a squatting or semi-seated position. When her labor becomes intense, the local village midwife, or a trusted grandmother, is called in. This indigenous midwife gives advice and comforts the family, often letting nature take its course. Berggren et al., (1983) reported that TBAs almost never performed vaginal or rectal examinations.

If the date of the delivery is anticipated early, the expectant mother remains at home indoors for several days. Teas, potions and baths may be administered. Care is taken to make sure that air does not enter the room where the women is awaiting delivery. Berggren notes that "in homes where 'voodoun' is practiced, there is a superstition about having much "light" on the subject, and midwives have recounted performing the entire delivery, even to cutting the umbilical cord, underneath a sheet" (Berggren et al., 1983:80). However, our respondents generally said it was important for the mother and the child to avoid catching cold, hence the need to keep openings in the room covered or closed.

Most women wish to be assisted by a *matrone* who, in fact, attends most deliveries. The *matrone* provides advice, gives massages using castor oil when appropriate, and seats the women on mats or a special round piece of wood used for delivery *(choukèt)*. Sometimes a low bed is used, with the women's back leaning against cushions and pillows while her husband or a close relative holds her arms.

When a child is being delivered, the midwife tries to make sure that everything goes normally and that the child emerges head first. Certain *matrones* put a wooden spoon in the mother's mouth which is suppose to make sure that it remains open, thereby providing the infant with sufficient air. Sometimes the midwife takes the baby's head in her hands and lowers it carefully so the shoulders and arms can come out. The newborn infant is then gathered up in a towel, a sheet, or a special apron. Use of an apron has been the custom since the colonial period (Moreau de Saint Mèry, 1958) as well as in 17th and 18th century France (Gelis, 1976).

Observing childbearing practices in the mid-1960's, Marshall noted that "the umbilical cord is cut with whatever is handy (raxor, knife, machete, scisors, piece of glass, sharp pieces of rock or metal) and by whomever happens to be about. When cords are tied, rags, thread, old string, or a grass are generally used. Cultural habits in rural Haiti dictate that something must be done to the cut end of the cord . . . The most frequent substances put on the cord end are powdered or crushed charcoal, burned strands of the straw bed mat, nutmeg and candle grease" (Marshall, 1968:69).

Our recent interviews suggest that more attention is given now to carefully cutting the cord. The *matrones* noted the importance of using a clean, unused raxor blade and waiting until the blood flows out of the cord and it is thin before cutting it.

Training of Traditional Birth Attendants

Efforts to train traditional birth attendants (TBA's) have been underway in Haiti in order to improve the survival chances of pregnant women and their off-springs since at least the 1950s. This training is expected to have two basic positive outcomes. First, the TBA's are expected to better perform deliveries through having learned about the importance of proper hygiene and procedures to follow during and after labor. They should also help women detect widespread health problems such as fever, anemia and tuberculosis, and give advice on proper nutrition during pregnancy, participate in pre and post natal clinics, and encourage women to use health facilities for family planning and other health needs.

With these goals in mind, the Division of Family Hygiene began a training program for Traditional Birth Attendants (TBA's), also called *matrones*, in 1976). A training manual and course were prepared. The reported number of *matrones* certified after a 3 month-training period, of one hour per week, were 8200 during the period from 1976–1983 (Division of Family Hygiene, 1984). It is estimated that there are about 11,000 *matrones* in Haiti, that is about 1 per 500 women.

Unfortunately, statistical reporting of births is incomplete in Haiti so that it is difficult to get an exact idea of program impact. However, in 1981, according to the Division of Family Hygiene's annual report, there were 36,150 deliveries in health facilities, 23,871 in Port-au-Prince and 21,279 in the rest of the country. Thus, almost 20 percent of the estimated deliveries in Haiti in 1981 took place in medical facilities. In addition, trained and certified *matrones* reported delivering 25,690 children in 1981, and additional 15 percent of the estimated total national deliveries. Thus reported coverage by trained personnel was 34 percent, an increase from 30 percent in 1979 and 32 percent in 1980.

Perhaps one of the most important accomplishments of the *matrones* training program is the impetus it has given to pregnant women to seek prenatal care. In a study done by the Division of Family Hygiene (DHF) in 1975 in the Jacmel area, most of the 75 *matrones* interviewed gave no prenatal care and were called upon only when labor began. In our more recent interviews in 1981–1982, all trained *matrones* referred women for prenatal visits. Similarly, Nalder (1982) found that the *matrones* in the Arniquet community health project area stressed the importance of prenatal visits.

In their pioneering work on eradicating tetanus in rural Haiti Berggren et al., found declines in neonatal tetanus based on various program activities. They note that in the 1956–1962 period, which witnessed both hospital treatment for tetanus and training of TBA's by Albert Schweitzer hospital nurses, there was a reduction in neonatal tetanus in their study area by 60 percent, from 220.5 to 136.9 deaths per 1000 live births. They believe that the training of indigenous mid-wives helped cause this decline in neonatal tetanus, evident in the 6 year period (Berggren et al., 1983).

More research is necessary to adequately assess the impact of TBA training on pregnancy outcome in Haiti. Nevertheless, it is clear that prenatal care is becoming common throughout the country. Service statistics from health centers all over the country indicated that in 1982 over 50 percent of pregnant Haitian women (about 105,000) were receiving prenatal care; they averaged two consultations per women. Progress has been impressive since less than 2 percent of women had access to prenatal care in 1974, less than 9 percent in 1975, and less than 19 percent in 1976. A major expansion of pre-natal visits has thus accompanied the expansion of the *matrone* program which has undoubtedly contributed to this movement.

Some Cost and Administrative Consideration of the TBA Training Program

The cost of the *matrone* training in salaries, supplies and materials used between 1977 and 1982 was $69,500, about $11,600 per year and less than $10 per matrone certified. This seems relatively small for the advantages the program has brought. Some of the current problems are due to the fact that an adequate system of supervision has not been developed, supplies often do not reach the TBAs in a timely fashion, and record keeping on the number of deliveries and their out-comes are incomplete. In addition to Division of Family Hygiene reports which raise these issues, Nalder (1981) looked into the structure of health personnel in Haiti and noted that by discontinuing training of nurse midwives at the Medical School in 1976, an important gap in supervision of *matrones* and other grassroots, outreach medical personnel has been created. She believes that "the nurse-midwife should be part of a health manpower pyramid which includes a large majority of nurses, auxiliaries, and *matrones . . .* The nurse-midwife, if properly trained in the public health aspects of MCH (maternal and child health), has the inherent commitment to the health of mothers and babies which is not found in any other category of health personnel, whose interest are broader . . . She is therefore invaluable to MCH program management in a system which delegates responsibilities to auxiliaries, *agent de santé*, and *matrone*" (1981:13).

Physicians tend to see improvement in maternal and child health by the increasing number of hospital deliveries. However, delivery in medical facilities is by no means a panacea for reducing maternal mortality and improving the survival chances of infants given current conditions. Haitian medical facilities are poorly supplied, seriously overcrowded and understaffed in urban areas, and often lack the most simple needs such as antiseptic solutions, cotton, even water.

In 1981, maternal mortality in Haitian medical facilities was over 350 per 100,000, ten times the rate in developed countries. Further, occupancy of maternity beds in health facilities outside of Port-au-Prince has been less than 40 percent for the 1975–1981 period. These facts suggest a multiplicity of problems that mean that in the foreseeable future, TBAs will have a major responsibility for assisting with child birth in Haiti, especially in rural areas.

Discussion

A disproportionally large body of literature on traditional religious practices exists and may lead one to believe that it will be extremely difficult for rural Haitians when faced with health issues to escape the heavy weight of traditional practices. Some even argue that "only by integrating the folk beliefs and customs into a modern system of treatment will any success be achieved in raising the health standards of the people of this country . . . By cooperating with the voodoo priests, western medicine can take advantage of the therapeutic potential inherent in voodoo practices" (Kiev, 1966:15). In fact, this does not seem to be true. When modern methods of health care become available, as has been the case especially in the last decade, Haitians are quick to accept and use appropriate technologies and modern medical care, without recourse to voodoo priests. For example, modern contraceptives have been well received by even rural, illiterate populations when made liberally available, and oral rehydration therapy has been found to be perfectly acceptable to both urban and rural mothers after a minimum of health education (Allman, James, 1982).

Based on in depth detailed analysis of reactions to an anthrax epidemic, Coreil summarizes Haitian behavior in regard to health problems as follows: "Routine natural illnesses are first treated with home remedies; if these fail the dispensary or leaf doctor is consulted. The latter two treatment options have comparable prices . . . Any illness which fails to respond to dispensary treatment after an extended time becomes supernaturally suspect and is dealt with accordingly" (Coreil, 1980:43). Superstition and magical practices are resorted to, above all, when modern medicine cannot provide results. Given the severly limited resources and often extremely difficult conditions confronting health personnel, it is not surprising that health institutions cannot provide satisfaction in many cases. Therefore, Haitians resort to traditional methods, *faute de mieux*.

The success in training *matrones* over the last 10 years supports the idea that important changes that improve the life chances of those most in need, can be made by the introduction in Haiti of low cost, relatively simple technologies. Social scientists have an important role to play in this process. They bring the analytical and methodological skills to assist with both the on-going, continuous process of monitoring, evaluation and operations research which can help programs improve, as well as the ability to assist often overly burdened health planners and administrators assess the long term impact of their policies and programs. To be more than just a vain slogan, "health for all" will require major inter-disciplinary efforts by social researchers, health personnel and communities directly concerned in the years ahead.

Conclusion

Cost data suggests that the program of training traditional birth attendants in modern preventitive health care is an inexpensive way of improving the life chances of poor rural mothers and their children. The enthusiastic acceptance of training by indigenous midwives, and the positive response by rural mothers, suggest that pessimistic arguments by some social scientists about the "traditional" mentality of rural people in Haiti needs to be reconsidered. The findings of this survey shows that simple, appropriate primary health care interventions, when carefully introduced, can be easily accepted by rural people. The potential for basic primary health care interventions is great and much can be done even with very limited resources. To help achieve this potential, social scientists interested in health issues in Haiti in particular, and developing countries in general, could usefully devote more effort in assisting in applied public health activities and encourage the intergration of modern and traditional practitioners.

References

Allman, James (1983) "Fertility and Family Planning in Haiti". Studies in Family Planning 13, 8/9: 237–245.

Allman, James, Jon Rohde and Joe Wray (1985) "Les conditions de succès d'un programme sélectif de soins de santé en pays en développement." Chapter 7 in Proceedings of IUSSP Seminar on Social Policy, Health Policy and Mortality Prospects, Paris, France.

Allman, Suzanne (1983) "Etudes ethnolinguistique de la lexique de la fécondité et la maternité en creole haitien." Unpublished doctoral disertation, University Aix-Marseille, France.

Berggren, Gretchen Glode, Adeline Verly, Nicole Garnier, Douglas Ewbank, and Wooly Dieudonné. (1983) "Traditional Midwives,

Tetanus Immunization and Infant Mortality in Rural Haiti." Tropical Doctor 13(79): 79–87.

Coreil, Jeannine (1980) "Traditional and Western Responses to an Anthrax Epidemic in Rural Haiti." Medical Anthropology (1): 79–105.

Division d'Hygiene Familiale (1984) "Evaluation du programme d'entrainement des matrones de 1979 à 1982." Port-au-Prince, Haiti.

Gelis, J. (1976) "L'accouchement au XVIIIeme Siècle." Ethnologie Française 6 (3/4): 325–340.

Nalder, Susan (1981) "An inquiry into the need to re-institute the training of nurse-midwives in Haiti." Port-au-Prince, USAID

Nalder, Susan (1982) "Analyse du fonctionnement du programme des matrones à Arniquet (District des Cayes)." Division d'Hygeine Familiale, Port-au-Prince.

Kiev, Ari (1966) "Obstacles to Medical Progress in Haiti." Human Organization 25: 10–15.

Marshall, F. (1968) "Tetanus of the Newborn, with Special Reference to Experiences in Haiti, W.I." Advances in Pediatrics 15: 65–110.

Moreau de Saint Méry. (1958) La Partie Française de Isle Saint-Domingue. Paris, La Rose.

Simpson-Herbert, Mayling, Phyllis T. Piotrow, Landa J. Christe and Janelle Streich. (1980) "Traditional Midwives and Family Planning." Population Reports J-22.

CHAPTER 5

Convenience, Cost and Courtesy: Factors Influencing Health Care Choices in Rural Morocco

Susan Schaefer Davis

Data is presented on health care options for people in a town of about twelve thousand in north central Morocco. Several cases of how traditional or modern options were chosen are described, and the reasons for these choices are compared to those for American populations. It is suggested that, in spite of the diverse cultural settings, similar factors are involved.

Factors Influencing Choice: The U.S.

IN MOST PARTS OF THE DEVELOPING WORLD, BOTH TRADI- tional and modern types of health care are available. An understanding of what each of these options involves and what leads to the choice of one over the other is essential for those concerned with health care delivery. Much of the research on factors influencing health care delivery however has been done in the United States and other western countries. That research suggests that specific factors such as convenience,

59

cost and courtesy influence the choice between modern and traditional health care, or lead to the underutilization of modern health facilities.

In the United States, Hines (1972) found that some American blacks will first consult local healers and paraprofessionals, and only approach the official health care system when these fail. In a study of black folk healers in Chicago, Snow (1978) points out that these healers have many positive characteristics: they treat the patient as a whole instead of focusing on isolated symptoms, charge less than M.D.s, and are more locally available to the poor. These traditional healers, like the Mexican-American *curanderos* studied by Moustafa and Weiss (1968), combine the natural and the supernatural in their diagnoses and treatments.

Like in third world countries, there is also underutilization of modern medical care facilities by the poor in the U.S.A. Dutton (1978, 1979) found three reasons for low use of such modern health facilities. In her study of poor families in Washington D.C., she hypothesized that these families used less medical care than they actually needed because of (1) cultural values, in which they less readily defined themselves as ill or had less faith in medical treatment, (2) insufficient financial coverage, and/or (3) a systems barrier. The latter means it is difficult for poor patients to locate and travel to the service they need, and that on arrival they may find it impersonal and feel uncomfortable. She concluded that this last factor is the most important. The first factor has some weight, but Medicaid has made the financial aspect relatively unimportant. Strauss echoes her feelings: "The poor, with their meager experience in organizational life, their insecurity in the middle class world, and their dependence on personal contacts, are especially vulnerable to [this] impersonalization" (1970:14). Dutton's findings, based mainly on blacks, were duplicated in a study of whites in Michigan (Rundall and Wheeler, 1979), in which they found the same three factors having the same orders of importance. These explanations will be evaluated in the Moroccan context.

Factors Influencing Choice:
The Moroccan Case

Background

   Described are health care choices made by people in a town of about twelve thousand in north central Morocco. Morocco shows the influence of African, European and Arab culture, with the latter dominant. The town of Zawiya (a pseudonym) is situated on a rich agricultural plain and enjoys a California climate, with hot dry summers and cool winters. The people are Muslims, and nearly all have Arabic as their native tongue. Zawiya is an excellent site to examine health care practices because of its intermediate position: it is neither an isolated rural community, nor is it fully urban. Many third world people live in such settings; they have access to modern medical care, but are still close to their own traditions. This is certainly true for Zawiya, where people's choices include a dispensary in town, a hospital in Kabar (the nearby market town of about forty-five thousand), or various traditional healers who live nearby.

   The data was collected by the participant observation method. Although local doctors, nurses and midwives were interviewed, the information presented here comes primarily from contact with the townspeople during the authors five year stay in that area, observing their experiences with both modern and traditional medicine. It became apparent that both economic and sociological factors made access to modern medicine difficult for the people, so that they usually tried the traditional cures, ("Muslim medicine") first.

Local Health Care Facilities: Modern

   Morocco built a modern health system during the period of French colonization (1912–1956), and has maintained it as the official system after Independence (Paul, 1975). There are two small medical dispensaries located right in Zawiya. One is government-operated and staffed by two male nurses, who provide limited care for minor injuries like cuts and administer injections prescribed and purchased in the larger town. They also serve as a referral agency, sending people with more serious problems to the hospital or a dispensary in town. The other local dispensary is operated by the Red Crescent (the Muslim Red Cross). It is staffed by one male nurse who gives injections purchased elsewhere; he may also provide advice on health questions. Thus in an emergency, local people can easily walk to a dispensary (the town is quite compact) and get the advice of trained nurses. In addition, a program begun locally in 1985 sends three paramedics door-to-door to give advice on child health and birth control; they give the pill to those who desire it and have been screened.

The larger town of Kabar, only two kilometers away, provides a much wider range of medical services. The main facility used by local people is the government hospital, offering both inpatient and outpatient care. There are a head doctor and two or three interns, several nurses, and three midwives. The town also has two large government-run dispensaries, operated by nurses, which treat less serious cases than the hospital. They dispense a variety of medications on doctor's orders, including birth control pills, and hold mother-infant nutrition classes. All these services are provided by the government at a minimal charge, or free if one has a certification of poverty from a local official.

For those able and willing to pay more, the larger town also has several private sources of health care. There are about four private doctors, mainly in general practice, but one is a cardiologist and another a gynecologist. There are several dentists who mostly do extractions and make false teeth, but some also fill cavities. Finally, there are several pharmacies selling a wide variety of drugs, many without prescription. This sometimes leads people to avoid the expense of a visit to a private doctor or the wait at the government hospital, and go directly to the pharmacist for treatment. For example, the pharmacist may give a man with an infected cut a penicillin shot and tell him to return in two days if it is not better.

Finally, for serious illness, cases needing surgery, or accidents, people may be sent to the provincial hospital about sixty miles away, or may seek private care in the capital. Some towns even had acupuncture available from visiting Chinese practitioners.

Local Health Care Facilities: Traditional

In contrast to the modern facilities, almost all the varieties of traditional care are available in Zawiya. If someone is not cured by the local person they consult, they may go to someone in another town who they have heard is especially effective, but s/he will be the same type of practitioner. There are many midwives in Zawiya, who assist at routine deliveries and sometimes know cures for sick babies and children. Most women practice folk medicine, in which they know herbal treatments for minor family illnesses. Other practitioners go beyond physical treatment and add a supernatural aspect. Sorcerers and sorceresses may treat infertility with herbal or chemical means, or may use written or spoken spells or prescribed actions to cure the condition. The *fgi* or religious teacher is often consulted to cure sick children with an amulet. A *fgi* may also treat an adult with a regimen of special diet, prayer, and isolation from others.

Maroccan Islam varies in many areas, in that local saints are considered to have healing powers. Sidi (Saint) Qasm founded Zawiya over 300 years ago. His descendants are known for their ability to treat specific maladies. For example, their saliva is thought to be good to cure sores. They also set broken bones, make small cuts to bleed people, or use a hot iron for cautery. In addition to consulting descendants of saints as curers, traditional medical help may be sought by visiting the tomb of a deceased saint or a shrine where a holy person once sat.

With this range of choices, several reasons lead people to start with traditional care. First, it is available right in town, even though the larger town is close because convenience is important. Second, it is usually less expensive. For example, childbirth in the hospital cost about $25 in 1982, while one could give a town midwife a 'gift' of about $5. A visit to the *fqi* with a sick child may cost $0.30, while it costs $0.20 to ride to the town pharmacy, and $1–$6 for a prescription. A final reason that people use traditional care first is that the practitioners are their neighbors and they know they will be received graciously; this is less clear when dealing with strangers in town. However, people may use both traditional and modern treatment, often simultaneously, if they feel it will benefit them. The following cases provide examples of the factors involved in health care choices.

Health Care Choices: Childbirth

Traditional childbirth always involves one of the several local midwives. A woman usually uses the same one for all her children, who later treat the midwife almost as a relative in terms of affection, and also may send her small remembrances on holidays. Here we will describe Dunya (only pseudonyms will be used) to show the training and duties of a midwife.

While some midwives learn this skill from their mothers, others do not, and Dunya is one of the latter. Once as a young woman she was returning from the outdoor market and heard a moan from the brush. She found a woman giving birth and helped her, cutting the cord with a piece of stone or wood; she had no other tool with her. After that, she began to help other village women with births, and recently the portly grandmother delivered her hundredth baby.

When Dunya delivers a baby, she is usually assisted by the mother or sister of the pregnant woman. The helper supports the woman, who is seated on a low stool or cushion, from behind, and Dunya sits in front to receive the baby. After the baby is born, she cleans it, cuts the cord with a razor, and ties it with a thread. Some midwives feel that the bones are "loosened" by childbirth, and have the new mother lie on her side while they sit on her, working from feet to head, pushing the bones "back together".

The traditional midwife is highly valued in Moroccan society; her skills are essential and frequently used. We see the respect accorded her in the fact that when Dunya delivered her one hundredth baby she was said to have "made the Hajj". This refers to the pilgrimage to Mecca in Saudi Arabia and is something that all Muslims should do once in their lifetime if possible. Few local people can afford such a trip, and those that do, are highly honored. While Dunya is very poor and could never afford to go, it is felt that she has gained the same amount of respect in God's eyes by her one hundred deliveries.

Traditional midwives have other skills as well. Dunya diagnoses pregnancy, and also treats infertile women by "cupping" (tanliyya): she places a lit candle under a clay cup on various parts of the abdomen. As the candle is extinguished, it creates a vacuum and thus suction on the skin. This is felt to open certain internal passages to allow conception to occur. Another midwife supplements insufficient breast milk with mint and sugar "tea" for the newborn; she may use peppermint or thyme. She further noted that peppermint is good for a baby with stomach pain.

We also see in Dunya an example of how the traditional health care provider often goes beyond dealing with physical or medical problems. In this instance, a local man was to appear in court to have his case decided. His family asked Dunya to borrow a client's baby's first shift for them; she could do so because people trust her not to misuse the special power associated with such a garment. She obtained the shift and the man carried it in court, because it is felt that God favors people who have such a garment.

Modern childbirth in the hospital in Kabar is also usually assisted by a midwife rather than a doctor. In this case the midwife, Ghazela, has had formal training in Casablanca. This is valuable because she often has to deal with more complicated deliveries, since most traditional women come to the hospital only for prolonged or especially difficult labors. Delivery in the hospital is done prone, which most women dislike but will accept. The midwife tells women to push when she sees they are ready, and she may also break the water or use chemicals to speed up labor; traditional midwives do not usually intervene so directly. After the delivery, women do not stay long in the hospital; they prefer to be home among their families.

Health Care Choices: Childhood
   Children in Morocco are highly valued, and both traditional and modern methods are uses to prevent and cure their illness.
   Much traditional protection of the child focuses on preventing ills caused by the evil eye. As in many Mediterranean lands, Moroccans believe people who envy a person can inadvertently harm them with a look. They also worry that compliments attract evil spirits. One can compliment a baby or child, but only after saying *"Tbarek Allah"* (the same as the "God bless" of many Italian-Americans), which serves to protect the baby. People may further protect a child by having it wear amulets, which often contain verses of the Koran written by the local religious teacher.
   There are various traditional treatments for a sick child. S/he may be taken to the religious teacher to get an amulet. Mothers also know herbal remedies for various illnesses. like a tea of *zaatar*, a thyme-like plant, to relieve stomach cramps. Many of the traditional cures involve the supernatural, calling for a visit to a saint's tomb, or physical contact with esteemed objects.
   Modern means of protection are also available through the government's free childhood immunizations. Infants born in a hospital are vaccinated against tuberculosis, and mothers are told to return soon for oral polio vaccine. However, since the majority of births are at home few children are reached in this way. Even mothers who were told to return never followed through on the polio series; perhaps the importance was not clearly explained, or it was too much of an effort to get into town at the right times. These problems were dramatically illustrated in the experience of a young woman who took her preschool niece and nephew to get their childhood immunizations.

The first step was to find out whether the injections were available free and where to get them. Amina went to one of the hospital doctors in Kabar, who told her the children needed a written slip from her. Amina requested the slip, but was told to return with the children to get it. Four days later, Amina brought the children. She got the slip and was directed to the larger town dispensary where the shots are given. En route, she met the male nurse she was to see, and he said the shots were only given on Monday and Tuesday; since it was a Friday, she had to return the next week.

Amina's third trip was about three weeks later; she had been delayed because her nephew had been ill. She went on a Tuesday, but was told to return the following Monday. On Monday morning Amina took the children to town and was told they only did shots in the afternoon. When she said she was just told "Monday" last time, the male nurse curtly remarked she must have had tar in her ears; she felt angry to be embarrassed in front of the other patients.

That Monday afternoon, on their fifth trip, the children finally got their TB tests. Amina had to take them back on Wednesday to get them read, and find out whether they could receive the other four DPT shots. Her experience discouraged Amina from pursuing immunizations.

Thus although the government provides free immunizations, many obstacles stand in the way of their use. These include the cost and logistics of transportation, the need for several visits for even one injection, and the fear of how one will be dealt with in a culture that stresses dignity. Moroccan sociologist Fatima Mernissi (1978) also found the latter problem, noting Moroccan paramedics often spoke French or literary Arabic to their uneducated female clients to stress the difference in their social classes.

Sick children seldom receive modern medical care from a doctor unless they are seriously ill or injured. Since no doctors have offices in the smaller town, a visit is inconvenient, but the main factor is the cost. Even with the free medical advice available at the hospital, a child ill enough to be taken will nearly always require medication, some of which may have to be bought. With a private doctor, there is in addition the fee of at least $5. It is common for a doctor to prescribe $15 to $40 of medication for a patient (child or adult); many people know they cannot afford this so do not go at all. Others, too shy to tell the doctor they cannot afford it all, randomly buy two of five medications and see if they work.

An example of both types of medical care for children is provided by the family in which the youngest daughter, Saida, had been plagued by itching skin for weeks; several attempts at herbal cures did not work. She was finally taken to the doctor, who diagnosed her condition as scabies and prescribed three medications. In addition, her mother was told to wash all the clothes and bedding—no mean task in a household of eight children, no washing machine, and no running water. The treatments were followed and the girl recovered fully. However, soon her brothers of 10 and 12 were complaining of itching and sores. One would assume that since the daughter had recovered so well, the family would return to the doctor. Instead, the boys were taken to a nearby saint's tomb beside a sulphurous spring, said to be good for skin problems. Although they bathed in this, the itching persisted. Both the expense of the visit and medication and the inconvenience of washing all the linens led the family to choose the traditional course.

The circumcision of all male children, usually between the ages of three and seven, provides a recurring need for health care. Townspeople can have the operation done in the traditional way by a barber-surgeon in their homes, or take the child to the Kabar dispensary for a nurse to cut the foreskin under sterile conditions. Although the modern method is available nearby, few take advantage of this—why? Again, both price and convenience are involved, especially the latter. The traditional operation is done near or in the boy's home, after which he lies down immediately. Since almost none of the local households own cars, the boy would have to walk or be carried the 2–4 kilometers home from the hospital, or his family would have to rent a taxi. Further, a hospital circumcision may cost approximately $15–$20, while at home it would be about $5. For both these reasons, local circumcisions are usually of the traditional kind.

Health Care Choices: Adult Women

We will use birth control as the one example space permits of adult health care because it is useful in demonstrating problems found in other cases. Further, birth control involves the largest number of people with modern health care. Although few rural women attempt to limit births before having three or four children, then nearly all try either traditional or modern birth control.

There are many traditional ways of preventing unwanted births, suggesting this as a longstanding area of concern. One method is used at a wedding, and involves inverting and hiding the bowl in which the cosmetic *henna* was mixed. People believe that the bride will not conceive for as many years as the number of days during which she does not see the bowl. Another traditional method involves a woman's friend getting bread from the home of a third woman, who lives in a different area and is unknown to the first woman. The latter takes a few bites of the bread, then puts it where she won't see it until she wants to become pregnant; then she takes it out and eats a bit more.

It is interesting that these, and several other traditional methods, involve the woman not seeing the materials involved. This may suggest an ambivalence on women's part about limiting births in a culture where children are much wanted, and in which their labor is a great help to the family and traditionally cost little. If there *is* this ambivalence about birth control in the traditional realm, it may also help us understand some of the problems we find in acceptance and usage of modern methods.

Traditional forms of abortion also exist. One involves the plentiful and poisonous oleander plant, and another requires the pregnant woman to ingest a mixture containing sulfur. In contrast to traditional birth control, many abortions use herbal or chemical agents and may be quite dangerous.

Modern forms of birth control have been available in small-town Morocco only since the late 1960s. The author saw a dramatic increase in women's knowledge of them in only three years. In 1967, women wondered if birth control pills really existed. By 1970, with no public information campaigns, women knew of both pills and IUDs (intrauterine devices) as ways to prevent pregnancy, that they preferred the pills, and that if they missed days on the pill, they were likely to become pregnant. This demonstrated women's ability to pursue and absorb knowledge that mattered to them personally.

There are several modern options available to the local woman who wants to limit births. She can go to the hospital to be examined, and they may have an IUD inserted, or be given a slip for free birth control pills at the larger dispensary; she must pick them up every month during her period. Few women want the IUD; whether well-founded or not, they have heard too many stories of problems with them. Another source of pills for wealthier women is the pharmacy, where they can be purchased without a prescription for about $1.20 per cycle. A third source of pills is the Moroccan Organization for Family Planning, a private group which sends a van to Zawiya every three months. Until March 1982 they distributed pills free of charge, reaching many women who could not afford pills or get into town. However, needing funds for operating expenses, they now sell pills at the low cost of about $0.35 per cycle. Unfortunately, a woman must purchase three cycles at once, and for many $1.05 is too much. Many women expressed interest in another method they had heard about: an injection which lasts one or six months. These are sometimes imported from Spain, but the Moroccan government has not yet approved their safety. The fact they do not need to be taken daily nor purchased often is probably the basis of their appeal. Finally, although technically illegal, abortions by doctors are available and used by women who can afford the price of $100–$200.

Two examples of users of modern birth control will help the reader to understand the attitudes and the problems involved. The first was a woman in her thirties, married to a widower and raising his three children as well as the three she bore him in five years; at this point she decided to use modern birth control. She bought one brand of pills at the pharmacy (several are available), but found they made her dizzy and also "weakened" her heart. She then requested free pills at the dispensary, switching brands, a reasonable move because pills vary widely in the amount of hormone contained. Unfortunately, she had the same problems and thus went to a heart specialist, who advised her to stop the pills or endanger her health. She now has another child.

Another case was that of Mina, who had used the pill successfully for five years, ever since her fifth child's birth. She had no side effects to motivate her to stop. Yet when a neighbor said she need not take pills daily, but only after she had slept with her husband, she did so . . . and soon became pregnant (as did the neighbor). Mina wanted an abortion, her husband was older with little income and she also dreaded the extra work. However, her mother was opposed to an abortion. She felt it was killing a soul (although that is not a universally-held tenant in Islam), and stated the common belief that "each child that's born will be provided for." While Mina grumbled, in the end she had the child.

Implications for Health Care Planners

The above examples concerning birth control illustrate many general aspects of the uses of and problems with traditional and modern health care in Morocco. As with much of modern medicine, people eagerly try modern methods, but their full scale adoption is inhibited by various problems. A major barrier is whether people have easy access to the new methods. Access may be limited by even a minimal cost if the people are poor. Another limitation is the need to travel even a short distance for treatment; many women found monthly visits to get free pills hard to arrange. Others reported difficulty getting the pills once at the dispensary because of supply or staff problems. (It is hoped the VDMS program described in note 1 will overcome these cost and access problems.) With such difficulties, people often turn to traditional methods. Further, the patient's own state may limit her use of modern birth control. The first woman felt her health was impaired and stopped the pills. The second woman's problem was attitudinal; while she was ambivalent about having another child, she could not overcome a family member's objections to an abortion.

The local use of birth control also allows us to perceive interactions between traditional and modern methods of treatment. Traditional birth control often forbids women seeing the "active ingredient", perhaps indicating ambivalence about the matter. This helps practitioners understand why local women say they would prefer long-term injections to daily pills.

In spite of wide cultural differences, we find several of the factors which determine how some Americans seek medical care are also relevant for many traditional Moroccans. The Moroccan data support Cockerham's statements that "The effects of time, energy, effort and distance have . . . been found as significant barriers to physician utilization . . ." (1982:90), and that ". . . the social organization of services is another factor highly related to help-seeking behavior" (1982:100). These refer to what Dutton (1978, 1979) called the systems barrier, which she and others have found inhibit the use of medical services by some Americans. Dutton's other two explanations for low usage are also relevant in this Moroccan setting; cultural views of illness may lead people to a traditional healer first, and the higher cost of modern treatment excludes many potential users. The financial aspect is more important in Zawiya than in America; in both cases there is governmental aid, but the systems barrier makes it more difficult to obtain for most Moroccans. These conclusions underline the importance of both an awareness of traditional health care practices and a user's view of how modern health facilities operate in understanding why people seek or do not seek a certain type of help.

References

Cockerham, William C. (1982) *Medical Sociology* (Second Edition). Englewood Cliffs, NJ: Prentice-Hall.

Davis, Susan S. (1983) *Patience and Power: Women's Lives in a Moroccan Village*. Cambridge, MA: Schenkman.

Dutton, Diana B. (1978) "Explaining the Low Use of Health Care Services by the Poor: Costs, Attitudes or Delivery Systems." *American Sociological Review* 43:348–368. (1979) "Patterns of Ambulatory Health Care in Five Different Delivery Systems." *Medical Care* 17:221–241.

Hines, Ralph (1972) "The Health Status of Black Americans: Changing Perspectives." Pp. 40–50 in E. Jaco (ed.), *Patients, Physicians and Illness*. New York: Free Press.

Mernissi, Fatima (1978) "Historical Insights for new Population Strategies: Women in Pre-Colonial Morocco; Changes and Continuities." Mimeographed paper sponsored by UNESCO, Division of Applied Social Sciences.

Moustafa, A. Taher, and Gertrud Weiss (1968) Health Status and Practices of Mexican-Americans. Advanced report II, Mexican-American study project. Los Angeles, CA: University of California.

Paul, James A. (1975) "L'organisation de la Sante et les Medecins apres L'Independence." *Review Lamilif* 69:18–26.

Rundall, Thomas G. and John R. C. Wheeler (1979) "The Effect of Income on use of Preventive Care: An Evaluation of Alternative Explanations." *Journal of Health and Social Behavior* 20:397–406.

Snow, Loudell F. (1978) "Sorcerers, Saints and Charlatans: Black Folk Healers in Urban America." *Culture, Medicine and Psychiatry* 2:69–106.

Strauss, Anselm I. (1970) "Medical Ghettos." Pp. 9–26 in Anselm I. Strauss (ed.), *Where Medicine Fails*. Chicago, IL: Aldine.

CHAPTER 6

Family Planning in Pakistan

Christiane I. Zeichner

Family Planning in Pakistan is an extensive administrative, multi-disciplinary technical program, educational movement and health service with the twin objective of population planning and economic development. Implementation of family planning programs within six Five Year Plans has advanced knowledge of communication, community involvement and motivation of target couples. Obstacles in the development of birth controlled population planning are discussed.

Introduction

THE POPULATION COUNCIL (1982) REPORTS FOR THE 134 Third World countries in 1982, that 72 officially support family planning programs and that 94 percent of the total Third World population lives in countries that officially support family planning to reduce population growth.

The most recent medium projections of the United Nations (1981) suggest that the population of the Third World will increase by 1.8-billion and than by another 2.0 billion, with the total growing from 3.0 billion in 1975, to 4.8 billion in 2000, to 6.8-billion in 2025. These projections suggest that without dramatic changes in either fertility or economy, or both, increasing numbers of people will live in poverty and deprivation in Third World countries during coming decades (Hernandez, 1985). Proponents of the view that population growth is a major cause of poverty in Third World countries emphasize that the fundamental demographic determinant of this rapid population growth is the sustained decline in mortality. Hence, they urge a demographic solution to the problem, namely public policies that will reduce aggregate fertility to levels commensurate with contemporary mortality (Bayles, 1980).

Dynamics of Population Growth in Pakistan

Pakistan's population, like those of other developing nations, has rapidly expanded in the last 35 years. In 1947, at its creation, Pakistan had a population of 32.5 million. The 1981 Census put the population at 84.3-million, which is estimated to have increased to about 1-billion in 1986. Pakistan is now the ninth most populous country in the world, with one of the highest annual growth rates. This rapid rate is burdened by a high dependency load (children). According to the 1981 census, 45 percent of the population are under 15 years of age, compared to 25 percent in western countries; 51 percent are between the age groups of 15 and 64 years, while only 4 percent are composed of persons over 65 (Pakistan, 1984). Of those 13 million who have received some education, 600 thousand have degrees from universities. Pakistan's population is predominantly Muslim (90 percent), rural (84 percent), and illiterate (85 percent). Approximately 45 percent of the total population resides in one-room housing units with an average occupancy of 6 persons per room, and the daily caloric intake per person remains below the average requirement of 2224. The incidence of malaria has decreased, but tuberculosis, a disease of poverty, can be found in one out of every 25 persons (Ministries-Division of the Government of Pakistan, 1981, 1984). Pakistan's high growth rate can be explained by a decline in mortality, due to better public health facilities and by advances and innovations in medical sciences. Likewise, public health measures have reduced large scale deaths from epidemics by mass inoculations, spraying against malaria, and elementary sanitation, all relatively inexpensive and easy to administer.

Three Decades of Family Planning in Pakistan

Programs designed to arrest population growth generally take long to yield any perceptable demographic impact, especially in developing countries like Pakistan where traditional values continue to promote pro-natalist attitudes and practices. The high population growth rate has become of great concern to the government. With the results of the 1951 Population Census, efforts to check its growth were initiated. The government set up five year time phases to bring growth rates to reasonable levels. During the first phase (1955–60) a token allocation of 500-thousand rupees (US $35 thousand) was made for family planning under voluntary auspices. During this phase the concept of *"Small Family"* was promoted and a few clinics were established in selected cities, but none in villages.

During the second Five-Year Plan (1960–65) family planning activities were initiated in the public sector, such as the work place. The need for the establishment of research centers and to bring fertility control to rural areas was recognized. With the allocation of 30.5-million rupees (US $2.5 million) it was hoped to reach 10 percent of the country's female population in child bearing age. The National Research Institute of Family Planning of Pakistan, and two American and two Swedish family planning research facilities were founded. Unfortunately, the second Five-Year Plan's targets were not achieved because (a) the monetary allocation was found to be insufficient to finance adequate supplies for distribution, (b) motivational barriers were tackled ineffectively, and (c) the program was administered as a regular function of

the health services, with a result that the already over burdened staff could not give further attention to family planning.

A breakthrough in the program came with the third Five
Year Plan (1965–70). Priority assigned to family planning can
be seen in the total initial budget of 284 million-rupees (US
$70 million) for the five year period. The goal for the program
was the reduction of the birth rate from an estimated 50 per
1000 annually to 40 per 1000, by reaching some 20 million
fertile couples. The administrative and organizational structure embraced about 100 thousand persons. Data shows that
between 1965 and 1968 some 2 million I.U.Ds were inserted,
600-thousand vasectomies performed and 371 million units of
conventional contraceptives were distributed. (Pakistan International Family Planning Conference, 1969). Despite excellent administration, this planning phase developed difficulties
soon after it was launched. The war with India resulted in
division of domestic resources from development to defense,
and reduction of foreign aid to Pakistan. This was followed by
drought in 1966 and floods in 1967 (Ministries-Division of the
Government of Pakistan, 1981).

Despite the shortcomings of the previous phase, the program strengthened family planning institutions. Emphasis
was put upon training of para-medical workers to create public
awareness of the importance of reduction of family size. Target
populations were approached by *"dias"* (indigenous midwives) for motivation and distribution of contraceptives at
their doorsteps. These "dias" became the chief instrument in
family planning programs. They contacted fertile couples,
distributed contraceptives, and attempted to motivate couples
by assurances. In 1969 there were approximately 50-thousand
"dias" operating in Pakistan; they worked on a part-time basis.
(Ministries-Division of the Government of Pakistan, 1970).

The need for motivation and education of target couples was
found to be the most important, but also the most difficult
task in family planning. Consequently, in the fourth phase
(1970–75), the administrative structure of the plan was re-
tained, and a new motivation strategy was used. This strategy
consisted of indigenous and western motivation techniques to

be described later in this chapter. Many indigenous part-time "dias" were replaced by full-time male and female motivators. Merely offering contraceptives to those unfamiliar with them, created new problems. It was found for example, that it was common practice for couples to alternate taking of oral contraceptives, the husband one day, the wife the next.

Because of the civil war between East and West Pakistan during the fourth phase in December 1971, much of the family planning field activities were suspended. Continuous internal political problems kept the program in a state of flux. In the fifth phase (1975–80), with the Islamisation of the country in 1977 the program became federalized and family planning activities were resumed in 1978. The new government in the sixth Five Year Plan (1980–85) relied primarily on community participation and involvement of local leadership to make the people recognize the need to reduce family size. In 1983, 243-million rupees (US $22 million) including foreign assistance, were spent on family planning. During this phase some 1250 family planning centers throughout the country provided planned parenthood advice, contraceptives and contraceptive surgery. The use of these centers is promoted by local influentials, who meet periodically to guide and support their functioning. Added were ten extension service teams to provide services and carry out contraceptive surgery, in camp situations, in Pakistan's remote rural areas. In addition 5000 feature films and documentaries on population reduction concepts were screened during this phase (Planning Commission of Pakistan, 1983).

Marketing the Concept of Family Planning to the Public

In the opinion of Berelson (1964) the main problem of family planning in developing nations is encountered at the communication level. To create motivation in the masses and to convey the concept of family planning, persuasive advertising must overcome conventional resistance to change. Good communication is vital. Couples have to be given strong motivation through which they will identify with and imploy means of limiting fertility, otherwise, contraceptive technology remains unused. While the relative availability and cost of different birth control methods may influence the decision of what technique to adopted to limit fertility (Hernandez, 1984), the consideration of time is another important factor in the dissemination process of ideas. Not only are psychological processes involved in the passage from one stage of decision making to another, but time is relevant in terms of the rate of spread of an innovation in a social system. The criterion for innovativeness is the degree to which an individual accepts a new idea earlier than others (Rogers, 1962). When accepting a new idea, an individual undergoes specific stages of decision-making. Bogue (1964), found when investigating dissemination of family planning concepts, that there are four identifyable stages through which a person goes: (1) awareness and interest, (2) information gathering, evaluation and decision to try, (3) implementation, and (4) adoption and continued use. Thus in order for a person to adopt a new idea s/he must be informed about it, must be motivated by internal and external sources to want to benefit, must believe in the credibility of the information, must perceive in social acceptance of the idea, and finally, must be able to link the use of the new idea to him/herself.

Western and Traditional Motivational Campaigns

The target individuals for family planning in Pakistan are a wife of fertile age with her husband, both of whom are usually illiterate. They customarily possess a traditional and religious outlook on life, and live in a rural area where the average age of marriage is 16 years, and where two thirds of marriages take place before the woman reaches 19 (The Family Planning Division, (1984).

A study conducted by the Family Planning Association of Pakistan (1974), investigated the effectiveness of two types of motivation methods: The western and the indigenous type.

Tested were the couple's knowledge, attitudes and practice of family planning. The investigators found that the three above mentioned variables were more likely to be increased by western motivation. Other findings were, that women were more receptive toward family planning, regardless of type of motivational campaign. Men, who in general showed less interest in reducing family size then women, felt more positively about western motivational techniques. Indigenous methods showed little effect on men.

Both, western and indigenous motivational techniques have become part of life in Pakistani villages and outskirts of urban areas. Indigenous methods make use of *"toliyan"* (village singers), puppet shows, colorful pushcarts, wall slogans, informal group meetings, local opinion leaders and home motivation by *"dias"* (local mid-wives) to every couple that asks for it. Puppet shows are organized by professional puppeteers, who speak local dialects and are employees of family planning organizations. Pushcarts decorated with colorful pictures and catchy slogans are pushed through the village during campaigns. In urban centers one can see permanently attached bill boards, approximately 20 feet high, and 10 feet wide, displaying a drawing of a couple with two children. In rural areas these bill boards show a couple with four children.

Western motivation techniques are based upon activities provided in informal, airconditioned family planning centers. Interested persons can view documentary films and slides; some five thousand of which were viewed in 1983. They can listen to tape recordings, look at posters, pamphlets, flash cards, documentaries, skits and songs presented on stage, and talk to motivators. Give-aways and the provision of clinical health services are another effective incentive for people to come and take a look (Kiani, 1981).

Islam and Family Planning

Family planning in Pakistan is an open topic among all walks of life. As discussed before, there is widespread public advertising, press coverage and backing of the country's President and other prominent leaders who encourage the adoption of the concept of "responsible parenthood and practice". Village store keepers were questioned how they felt about being asked by the government to sell contraceptives. Most of them were proud that their shops had been selected to help in the program in which the President attached such great importance (Planning Commission, 1983).

The large publicity of family planning activities has brought about sporadic opposition from Muslim religious groups. Islam has a general pro-natalist position, and opposition to the country's family planning program has been disseminated in forms of speeches in Friday prayer services. In order to have a dialogue with the religious community, the government of Pakistan sought the support of Muslim theologians in Pakistan and other Muslim countries who declared themselves in favor of family planning. Much of the opposition is directed against the government's support of the use of every tried method of contraception available to every couple that asks for it. This attitude worries the traditional Muslim religious community. It is feared that such values will lead to depopulation of the country and encourage sexual immorality (Shahidullah, 1978). According to some theologians, Islam does not forbid the temporary prevention of pregnancy, as long as the method of contraception is legal according to Islam, harmless, and voluntary. It is considered valid only in the following four circumstances: (a) To give a woman a chance to rest between pregnancies, (b) if either or both partners have a disease which can be transmitted to their offspring, (c) to safeguard the woman's health, and (d) if the husband's finances are insufficient to support more children (Sharabassi, 1978).

Conclusion

Pakistan has a carefully constructed, and frankly stated population policy. The government's policy is oriented to stabilizing the fertility rate on behalf of economic development and of raising the people's living standard. This policy was initiated with the first Five-Year-Plan in 1955. It calls for a large-scale program for reproductive health services, education, motivation for family planning, provision of birth control advice and contraceptives, and government supported research on demographic trends and contraceptive methods. Centers and clinics for family planning have been established in large numbers in rural areas, and are available at urban medical and health centers. Much research is done on how to make programs more effective, and United Nation teams share their expertise with the Family Planning Association of Pakistan.

Pakistan's family planning program has two useful and effective features. The first being, that family planning is treated as an interdisciplinary public relations activity rather than a clinical medical activity. Secondly, the program makes use of public as well as governmental opinion leaders in well organized programs, and efforts are based on motivating a psychologically resistant population. Family planning in Pakistan is consolidated with the health sector, mass media, other communication agencies and community development services.

Pakistan is a poor country with a population of 89 million. Approximately half of the population consists of people under 15 years of age, soon to start producing children themselves. Currently, less than 10 percent of the country's fertile couples are believed to practice contraception. Even if this figure was raised to the government's goal of 20 percent, no substantial difference in population would be made unless the contraceptive figure went up to a difficult to achieve 35 percent. Therefore, the mere distribution of contraceptives to target couples is not enough to lower population growth. Ways have to be found to motivate the poor, illiterate, tradition-minded population in rural areas, accustomed to having large families, to space and limit their children (Hernandez, 1984).

Results from the World Fertility Survey (Lightbourne and Singh, 1982) show that Pakistan belongs to those countries that have been relatively successful in achieving some immediate goal—the provision of supplies, services and information about modern birth control methods to women and couples. Now it is necessary to identify those programs that work and to understand why programs fail.

Although it is necessary to identify those programs that work and understand why others fail, family planners must now deal with the possible legal problems that may influence the availability of contraceptive supplies and jeopardize the development of new methods.

In the United States many modern methods of birth control have recently been plagued by increased litigation against pharmaceutical companies that manufacture them. These legal problems may have already influenced family planning policies of organizations such as U.S. Agency for International Development (A.I.D.). In the past A.I.D. granted support to any family planning program offering more than one method of birth control. Today, A.I.D. policy still makes available the widest possible range of birth control methods to couples of developing countries, but now has become the single, largest supporter of Natural Family Planning (NFP) training and research in the world (Johnson and Reich, 1986).

Presented at the 36th Annual Meeting of The Society for the Study of Social Problems, New York, 1986

References

Bayles, M. D. (1980) Morality and Population Policy: Tuscaloosa The University of Alabama Press.

Bogue, Donald (1962) Written Communication for Family Planning. Chicago, University of Chicago Press.

Family Planning Division. Government of Pakistan. (1984) Proposals of Family Planning Division for Family Planning Sector. Islamabad, Pakistan.

Hernandez, Donald (1984) Success or Failure? Family Planning Programs in the Third World, Greenwood Press. Westport, Connecticut. (1985) Fertility Reduction Policies and Poverty in Third World Countries: Ethical Issues. Studies in Family Planning and Urban Demography No. 4.

Johnson, Jeanette H. and Julie Reich (1986) The New Politics of National Family Planning. Family Planning Perspectives. Vol. 18, No. 6. Nov/December. The Alan Guttmacher Institute N.Y.

Kiani, Aquila (1981) Sociology of Development in Pakistan, Social Research Center, University of Karachi, Pakistan.

Lightbourne, R. and S. Singh (1982) The World Fertility Survey: Charting Global Childbearing. Population Bulletin 37 (1), Washington D.C.

Ministries Division of the Government of Pakistan (1970) Pakistan: An Official Handbook. (1981) Pakistan: An Official Handbook. (1984) Pakistan 1984: An Official Handbook Ministry of Information and Broadcasting. Barqsons Printers, Islamabad, Pakistan.

Pakistan International Family Planning Conference at Dacca (1969). Population Control: Implications, Trends and Prospects. Islamabad, Pakistan.

Planning Commission of Pakistan. (1983) Sixth Five Year Plan 1983–1988. Population Welfare: Correcting the Misdirected Investment, Chapter 21, Government of Pakistan. Islamabad, Pakistan

Population Council. (1982) Population and Family Planning Programs: A Compendium of Date through 1981, 11th Edition, New York.

Rogers, Everett (1962) Diffusion of Innovation, New York Free Press.

Shahidullah, Muhammad (1978) Family Planning and Islam. Muslim Attitudes toward Family Planning, The Population Council, New York.

Sharabassi, Ahmad (1978) Islam and Family Planning. Muslim Attitudes toward Family Planning. The Population Council, New York.

U.S. Department of State, (1985) Pakistan Background Notes. Pubn. No. 7748 Office of Media Services, Bureau of Public Affairs. Washington, D.C.; US Government Printing Office

CHAPTER 7

Health and Disease in Rural Ghana

Gabriel B. Fosu

Examined are how the people of Berekuso, a rural community in Ghana, view health and disease. Three main types of disease-causes are distinguished: Diseases caused by natural agents, supernatural agents and those caused by both, natural and supernatural agents. The cause of a disease was found to be the most important aspect of therapy.

Introduction

A CONTINUAL CHALLENGE TO THOSE WHO PLAN AND IM-plement health care programs in developing countries is the effective delivery of health care with limited resourses. One approach in improving resource allocation is the assessment of the factors that determine the use or non-use of health services for targeted populations such as rural dwellers. Studies indicate that the choice of which service to use and when, may not be random, but it may depend, among other things, on the health belief system (Gould, 1957; Foster, 1958; Colson, 1971). This suggests the need for each system to be studied in detail because the knowledge of a group's basic premise about health maintenance and illness etiology can assist health care programs and medical interventions. This chapter examines the effects of health beliefs on the use of health services in a village in Ghana. The discussion is seen as a contribution to the understanding of African systems of health and healing.

Description of the Study

The study was undertaken by the author in a traditional rural Ghanaian community, Berekuso, which had a population of 1243 in 1976 (Fosu, 1981). The investigator lived in the village for one year. Participant observation method was first used to gain an insight into the cultural practices and social behavior of the people. Then indepth informal interviews were done with knowledgeable people like the chief, fetish priests and herbalists who are regarded as repositories of tradition and are, therefore, influential in defining what is the proper behavior. Interviews using structured questionnaires were also undertaken in 60 randomly selected households out of 180 households to determine the health belief system. At the second stage of the household interview survey, a morbidity survey of the selected households was undertaken. A combination of techniques, including health logs, clinic records and health interviews were used to detect the illness episodes in the households.

Medical Systems

Berekuso is an agricultural village where the people live very close to nature and to the soil. Descent and kinship groupings are the basis of economic, political, religious and social organizations. It lies 25 miles northwest of Accra, the capital of Ghana. Even though there has been very little structural change in the village, contact with western society, and the introduction of modern institutions like clinics and schools have weakened some of the traditional belief systems. For instance, two medical systems, traditional and scientific, exist at the same time in the village. This means that alternative and often competing medical services are available to the people (Twumasi, 1975). Some components of each of the two systems will be discussed briefly.

Practically every adult in Berekuso knows of some herbs or recipes for the relief of common ailments, since medical knowledge is an aspect of culture that people learn during the process of socialization. Every family has its own favorite herbal prescriptions which have been proven over the years. These are kept within the lineage or family and are handed down to its members. The art of healing, therefore, becomes a family specialty.

However, healing is one of the most important roles in Berekuso society. Thus it is entrusted to competent and well-trained people. Great prestige is accorded those who occupy the status of healers in Berekuso, because they are regarded as people who have special qualities and whom the gods have chosen for the role of intermediaries. The calling to be a healer usually occurs at a very young age. Then, as Twumasi (1975) has most elaborately discussed, they undergo several years of intensive training and apprenticeship before they are allowed to set up independent practice.

Traditional healers in Berekuso may be divided into two major groups: *Akomfoo*, fetish priests and priestesses who are usually priests or diviners of certain gods or deities, and *Adunsifoo*, herbalists who use herbal medicine to treat diseases. Though both groups may practice a little of each other's trade, there is a tendency for each group to specialize. In addition to these two groups there are traditional midwives *awogyefo*, many of whom have had further training at the Danfa clinic.

Traditional healers use magico-religious symbols which have great meaning and significance for their patients. The symbols include particular styles of dressing, language and tools. Their technical knowledge includes healing procedures, mystical incantations and group singing. These symbols and techniques of healing are derived from theories about the

causes of diseases. They draw on a theoretical formulation
which is made up of religious, magical, philosophical and
social components. With this theory they are able to explain
the mysteries of why people get sick, why they recover or why
they die. There are five fetish priestesses and six herbalists of
whom three work as traditional midwives in the village of
Berekuso.

A major source of modernization at Berekuso is the introduction of the scientific medical system by the Danfa Comprehensive Rural Health and Family Planning Project (Danfa
Project). The Danfa Project has developed satellite clinics by
means of which health services are taken closer to the village
populations. People in and around Berekuso have access to
such a satellite clinic which is run every Monday at Berekuso.
Its introduction has given rise to new sets of interests and
values that are often regarded as imcompatible with, and a
threat to traditional theories of disease and medical practices.
When scientific medicine, therefore, comes to a rural area
like Berekuso, it usually comes both as a strange and perhaps
fearful innovation, and as a competitor of established ways of
obtaining help for the sick. Thus, even though its introduction
has helped to broaden the cultural experience of the rural
dwellers, it has also brought some problems to the people in
their pursuit of medical care. This will be examined further in
subsequent sections.

Definition of a Health State

When the respondents were asked to define disease, they
made a clear distinction between good health and disease.
Operationally defined, disease was anything that the respondents labelled as *yadee*, meaning sickness, illness and morbidity. Disease was seen as a natural consequence of man's
relationship with his physical and social environment. In response to the question, "What do most people mean when
they say that they are sick?", 46.8% of the respondents answered when specific symptoms of physical condition are
present, 34% said when they generally feel weak and unwell,

and 4.9% said when, as a result of their normal duties. Only 1.6% answered when a condition that kills is present. The rest were combinations of the first three responses.

An analysis of the disease classification system was undertaken to determine the impact of social change on traditional medical beliefs and practices. It was found that the foundation of the disease classification system is what is believed to be the cause of a disease, because, whether treatment should begin at all, and if so which remedies should be sought depend on what is thought to be the cause of the disease. However, in determining the cause of a disease they take into account several factors: the events in the life of the sick person which might explain the onset of the disease; the severity of the disease; the type of people who are known to be susceptible to that particular disease as well as the number of people who are affected by the same disease at the same time.

In order to get a deeper insight into the system of disease classification, therefore, 308 respondents in the Berekuso survey were asked to name any five diseases. They were then asked to classify these diseases according to what is believed to be the cause of each. The interviews yielded 1,532 responses dealing with 62 specific diseases (Fosu, 1981). About 47% of responses classified diseases as naturally caused, 39.3% as supernaturally caused, and 14.1% as both naturally and supernaturally caused (Diagram 1).

An attempt was made to determine the extent to which different individuals differ in the way they classify diseases. While several studies have amply documented cross-cultural variations in disease classification (Evans-Prichard, 1937; Field, 1960; Frake, 1961; Chen, 1970; Fabrega, 1971; Warren, 1974) much less is known about such differences within a single society. The following variables were studied: age, education, sex, religion and occupation.

Findings

The classification of disease by the age of respondents showed that the younger the individuals are, the more they

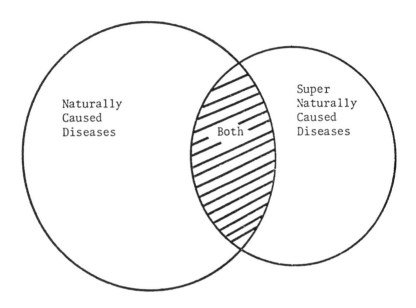

Diagram 1
DISEASE CLASSIFICATION SCHEME

are likely to show a scientific attitude towards diseases. Over 54% of all those below 30 years of age classify diseases in natural terms. Conversely, less than 40% of all persons above 30 years of age classify diseases as naturally caused. Disease causation according to educational level of the respondent showed that the classification of diseases in natural terms increases greatly with the level of education. While 33.1% of those with no formal education classify diseases as naturally caused, as high as 66.7% of respondents with secondary school education classify diseases as naturally caused. There is very little difference between respondents with primary and middle school education. However, the difference between respondents with elementary and those with post elementary school education is quite appreciable. Thus, the classification of diseases as supernaturally caused decreases with formal education (less than 32% in each category) classify diseases in supernatural terms. Several reasons may contribute to such differences in disease classification according to educational status and age. Education, like age, is associated with changes in attitude. The younger and more educated person is more likely to show a scientific attitude toward diseases, because formal education tends to weaken traditional cultural practices.

Slightly more females (48.2%) than males (44.7%) classify diseases in natural terms. This difference is very small (3.5%). The difference between the sexes with regard to supernaturally caused disease is even smaller (1.3%). One would have thought that females in Berekuso who have less formal education than males, would classify most diseases as supernaturally caused. A possible explanation for the reversed situation may be due to sexual differences in handling diseases within the household (Litman, 1974). As females, especially the wife-mother, deal with diseases in the household more often than males (especially with diseases of children), it is expected that they would more frequently come in contact with hospitals. Such contacts are likely to influence their attitudes towards diseases. Consequently, they may classify most diseases as being caused by natural agents.

Categorization of the causes of diseases was intimately linked to religion. While a majority of Catholics (60%), Presbyterians (67.3%), and Methodists (65.7%) classified most diseases as caused by natural agents, the greater proportion of Apostolics (53.5%), Moslems (55%), Traditionals/Pagans (57%), and Jehovah Witnesses (44.4%) classified diseases as caused by supernatural agents. The differences might be due to differences in religious beliefs.

Different occupational groups also classified diseases in different ways. About 52 percent of the farmers questioned classified diseases as supernaturally caused. This may be a reflection of their concept of the universe. Since they live very close to nature, and come in contact with many events which are difficult to explain in natural terms, they tend to have great respect for the unseen forces of nature. On the other hand, those in the clerical and lower professional occupations classified diseases mostly as caused by natural agents. This was expected because their jobs require some formal education, and exposure to western ideas. Also to legitimate the sick role and absence from work, those in clerical jobs are usually expected to go to the hospital or clinic.

Use of Traditional and Western Health Care

The pattern of use of the various health services in Berekuso was found to vary with the way individuals classify diseases. Berekuso clinic was used more by those who tend to classify diseases in natural terms, by the younger age groups, literates, females, Christians, and by clerical and professional workers. On the other hand, illiterates, farmers, Moslems, and others who followed more traditional religions relied very much on traditional medical services.

Almost all supernaturally caused diseases were treated within the context of traditional medicine (by traditional healers or by self-medication). In the few instances where supernaturally caused diseases were taken to the clinic, the people did so mainly for symptom relief, but they trusted the traditional healer to effect the actual cure. The efficacy of traditional medicine in treating supernaturally caused diseases was reinforced by reasons given by respondents. The majority of people who used traditional medical services did so mainly because of their effectiveness. Since naturally caused diseases could be treated either at the clinic or by traditional medicine, it is not surprising to note that some literates also used the services of traditional medical practitioners and family treatment. Berekuso clinic is open every Monday. Thus when clinic services are not available the next alternative may be either the traditional healer or self-treatment. In fact many people who used self-treatment said that they did so because it was the service most readily available at that time. The reported use of traditional medical practitioners was surprisingly low for a rural community. This may reflect the availability of the clinic, now that one has been made available in Berekuso.

The instances in which diseases are neither traditionally nor scientifically treated are still very high. This is surprising in a village with a modern clinic and several traditional medical practitioners. Actually, the rate of self-treatment was very high. This suggests, and supports the widely held view that the mere presence of a modern health facility in a community does not necessarily mean that people will use it (Polgar, 1962). One has to take into account other aspects like how clinics are organized and significant others in the family who are actively involved in the treatment decision making process. Actually, "advice" plays an important part in seeking medical care. When a person is sick at Berekuso it is the responsibility of those around him to decide how to get him cured. What to do at that time may depend partly on their knowledge of what is available, and partly on the advice they receive from people whose views they respect. In this regard, when respondents were asked, "Did you consult any member of your family before any action was taken on your illness?", the majority (59.6%) answered yes. Out of this group 17.7% consulted their mothers, 14.3% their spouses, 6.6% their fathers, 5.1% their grandparents, 3.6% their mother's brothers, and 3.1% their brothers and sisters. The reasons given for consulting these relatives ranged from advice (22.5%), permission (21.9%), to the fact that they were experts on the condition (4.1%). It was noted that utilization behavior differed with the people they consulted. "No treatment" cases, for instance, were highest when brothers and sisters were consulted.

Prevention of Illness

When respondents were asked, "Could you have prevented this illness?", 20.2% said yes, 75.5% answered no, and 4.2%

said they did not know. When they were asked the methods they would use to prevent diseases, several methods were mentioned. They may take positive steps to avoid predisposing conditions like exposure to excessive heat and cold, and to avoid all forms of contact with diseased persons which they believe make people vulnerable to some contagious disease. Those afflicted with leprosy, for instance, may be banished from the village to prevent other people from contracting it. Other positive forms of prevention may include drinking herbal medicines regularly. With regard to supernaturally caused diseases special efforts to prevent them may include living in harmony with relatives, and amicably settling all quarrels. Also, they may have to observe certain traditional norms and taboos such as not eating totemic animals in order to prevent the incidence of some diseases. Other measures may include the wearing of talismans and amulets, burning of incense and herbs, and the utterance of mystical words or incantations so as to ward off evil forces.

Since children are thought to be particularly susceptible to certain spiritually caused diseases their mothers take special precautions before and after birth to prevent them from such diseases. All these indigenous methods of prevention are logical corollaries of the concepts of disease causation. Spiritually caused diseases would have to be countered by equally spiritual but more powerful forces. Further research needs to be done to explore more systematically the indigenous concepts of prevention. The use of such indigenous concepts will then make attempts to change beliefs and behavioral patterns more efficient. These could also have important implications for the needed emphasis on preventative and public health programs.

The study also points to the fact that the people use the services of drug sellers to a certain extent. Drug sellers act as medical advisors for a wide range of illnesses. It may be worthwhile to consider further the potential role of travelling drug sellers in rural health care. The objectives of a rural health plan include preventive, curative, and educational promotive services. These presuppose that a minimal level of health care should be made available to everybody to enable him to achieve complete physical, mental and social well-being. Recent efforts to expand rural health care services have included the use of auxiliary health workers. Traditional midwives have been trained and volunteers have been recruited. Since travelling drug sellers are now meeting some of the needs of rural dwellers, especially where modern medical services are lacking, it might be worthwhile to use their services.

Cost of Health Care

The purchase of health services is like the purchase of any other commodity; it is determined by income and economic factors. The reality of economic barriers associated with poverty in developing countries is great so that even minimal charges may make the use of health care services prohibitive for the poor. In Ghana modern medical services are provided free by the government to most of the population. But for the very poor, the problem of obtaining modern medical care may be difficult as they live far away from the clinic.

In 79.3% of all reported illnesses no cost was involved. About 8.8% of reported cases involved costs less than 30 cents, 5.2% between 31–60 cents, 1.6% between 61–100 cents, 1.0% between 151–300 cents, and 4.1% involved cost more than three dollars. It is expected that where no treatment is sought, there should be no cost. This was the case with the 48 reported cases in which no treatment was sought. Approximately 91.7% of all cases taken to Berekuso clinic alone did not entail any costs, because services at the clinic are free. In the six cases where some cost was incurred, it was mostly on food, or on empty bottles to collect medicine, or on transportation. It is interesting to note that 81% of cases that were treated by self involved no costs. This may be due to the fact that those concerned prepared their own herbal medicines, and they had to buy some drugs only on a few occasions (19%). All other services used involved some expenses. Those who used the services of traditional medical practitioners and clinics outside Berekuso incurred costs ranging from one pesewa to more than three cedis. About 33.3% of cases exclusively taken to traditional medical practitioners were free, but in all other instances charges were involved. In some cases fetish priests do not charge their clients, and in others they wait until they are cured before they charge them. Traditional healers are by custom morally responsible to treat the sick and the poor. Thus it is inconceivable for a traditional healer to give inadequate attention or completely refuse care to a poor sick person.

Policy Implications

More research is needed, especially in rural areas to determine who in the kinship network decides where family members should go for treatment. The role of the family and its kinship network in influencing the choice of treatment has long been overlooked and several questions may be raised in this regard. For instance, are there certain diseases in which the members of the extended family play a more important role in defining, consulting, and referring, while in others noticeably fewer members are involved? Does the geographical proximity of the family and relatives affect the nature of its influence on utilization behavior? Is kinship involvement in any way related to the particular type of service being used? Does the family network affect the efficacy of care after a service has been utilized? The emphasis on the strategies that people in rural areas employ to cope with medical problems will help to make understandable some of the problems involving the delivery of health care that plague many developing countries and that are likely to continue in the future. By determining the people who influence the patient's choice of health care services, therefore, health educators can focus on certain target populations. This in the long run may increase the rate of utilization of health care services.

Summary

This study has shown that the people of Berekuso classify diseases into three main types: diseases that are caused by natural agents, those caused by supernatural agents, and those caused by both natural and supernatural agents depending on the social circumstances surrounding such illnesses. Disease classification varied with such socio-demographic factors as age, sex, education, religion and occupation. It is suggested that the perception of illness and the type of treatment used is influenced by formal education, new economic opportunities and one's experience or contact with urban communities. Evidence from the morbidity survey confirmed the experience in most developing countries regarding the simultaneous use of both traditional and modern medicine (Twumasi, 1975). It further indicated the persistent use of traditional medicine by the elderly group of the population. The knowledge of the cause of a disease allowed a fairly accurate prediction of what resources would be used. Supernaturally caused diseases were treated with traditional medical services, while the services of drug sellers and clinics were used in treating naturally caused diseases.

References

Chen, C. Y. (1970). "Classification and Concepts of Causation of Mental Illness in a Rural Malay Community." *International Journal of Social Psychiatry* XVI(3): 205–215.

Colson, A. C. (1971). "Differential Use of Medical Resources in Developing Countries." *Journal of Health and Social Behavior* 12, p. 226–237.

Evans-Pritchard, E. E. (1937). *Witchcraft, Oracles and Magic Among the Azande*. Clarendon Press, Oxford.

Fabrega, H. Jr. (1971). "Some Features of Zinacantecan Medical Knowledge," *Ethnology* 9:25–43.

Fosu, Gabriel B. (1981). "Disease Classification in Rural Ghana: Framework and Implications for Health Behavior", *Social Science and Medicine* Vol. 15B(4) pp. 471–481.

Field, Margaret J. (1960). *Search for Security: An Ethnopsychiatric Study in Rural Ghana*. Faber and Faber, London.

Frake, C. O. (1961). "The Diagnosis of Disease Among the Subanum of Mindanao." *American Anthropologist* 63:113–132.

Gillies, E. (1971). "Causal Criteria in African Disease Classification," (mimeo).

Gould, H. A. (1957). "The Implications of Technological Change for Folk and Scientific Medicine." *American Anthropologist* 59:507–516.

Litman, T. J. (1974). "The Family as a Basic Unit in Health and Medical Care: A Social Behavioral Overview." *Social Science and Medicine* 8:495–519.

Polgar, S. (1962). "Health and Human Behavior: Areas of Interest Common to the Social and Medical Services". *Current Anthropology* 3(April)pp. 159–205.

Twumasi, P. A. (1975). *Medical Systems in Ghana*. Tema: Ghana Publishing Co.

Warren, D. M. (1974). "Disease, Medicine and Religion Among the Techiman Bono of Ghana: A Study in Culture Change." Unpublished Ph.D. Dissertation, Indiana University.

CHAPTER 8

Voodoo and Santeria: Traditional Healing Techniques in Haiti and Cuba

William B. Harvey

Religious practices among the peasants of Haiti and Cuba strongly affect the attitudes that they hold toward modern health care delivery systems. The faiths of Voodoo and Santeria assist their adherents in maintaining both physical and psychological well-being in living conditions that are usually harsh and severe. As the descendants of former African slaves, peasants in both countries prefer using traditional practitioners to scientifically trained personnel for treatment of illness or infirmity. In shaping the frameworks and perspectives of the indigenous people, the cultural imperatives of the two countries and the general responsiveness to those concepts exemplify the necessity for health care planners to incorporate considerations of existing belief systems and value orientations in the design of effective health care delivery.

IN EXAMINING HEALTH SERVICES, PARTICULARLY IN Third World countries, the cultural framework must be carefully considered in order to gain an understanding of how the indigenous peoples view sickness, disease, and appropriate treatment methods. The particular examples of Cuba and Haiti, Caribbean island nations in the shadow of the United States, show how traditional values and attitudes can impact on the degree of acceptance and utilization of modern health care practices.

Perspectives on health care do not exist in a cultural vacuum. The views that individuals manifest are acquired in the context of enculturation, when in the process of their development and growth, the prevailing conceptualizations and ideologies of the larger culture are inculcated into the minds of the individual citizens. Haiti, almost exclusively, and Cuba, to a large degree, are populated by people of African ancestry, whose viewpoints are substantially affected by traditions and ideas that originate in the homelands of their ancestors.

Both the existence and significance of these African cultural traits among Blacks living in the Americas have been validated by anthropologists. Herskovits (1958) argues that these Africanisms have substantial impact on the perspectives held by Blacks in the Western Hemisphere, including those in Cuba and Haiti. Thus, the degree of their willingness to use modern health care services is affected by these considerations because, as Simpson (1978:299) observes, the "related magical rituals furnish the means of alleviating human problems."

Both Haiti and Cuba are poor, underdeveloped nations by Western standards. In both countries, the predominant values and conceptions have a traditional, rather than a Western orientation. In order to understand the viewpoints that Haitian and Cuban peasants hold in regards to health care, one must first understand the cultural dynamics of the two nations. Following is a presentation of the key issues related to the traditional Haitian and Cuban religions of

Voodoo and Santeria, and the effects of these two faiths on health care delivery.

History of Voodoo and Santeria

Voodoo and Santeria have histories that are somewhat similar. The development of Voodoo can be traced to the importation of African slaves in 1510 to the country that is now called Haiti. The African victims of the slave trade brought their religious convictions with them, but while the traditional beliefs of those slaves were unchanged as a result of their shift in location, they did have to perform their traditional rites and services in a disguised manner. The laws of the day prohibited the assembly of slaves for purposes other than Catholic worship, which was the religion of the masters. It is from the intermixture of religious concepts from the Dahomean, Senegalese, and Congolese tribes, combined with certain beliefs about Catholic saints, that Voodoo began to emerge.

The term *Voodoo*, or *Vodoun* is a "a Dahomean word which means God, protective spirit, or the 'company of gods' . . . Vodoun is a conglomeration of various African divinites with the further addition of the Christian Trinity, plus the roster of saints of Catholicism, all thrown together." Barrett, (1974:100) From Herskovits' (1937:139) perspective, Voodoo is "a complex of African belief and ritual governing in large measure the religious life of the African peasantry." As a belief system which combined historical conceptions with practices that were acceptable in a hostile social environment, Voodoo is a striking example of a cultural adaptive mechanism used by members of an oppressed group as a survival technique.

Generally speaking, religious ceremonies take believers away from the mundane affairs of life, sometimes by presenting exhilirating experiences. On such occasions, participants often dress in ceremonial or special clothing, sacred objects are prominently displayed, familiar and emotional songs are sung and well-known myths are recited. In Voodoo, when these ceremonial activities occur, they simultaneously serve two functions: some members of the faithful gain "understanding" through possession by a deity, ancestor, or spirit; and the entire gathering reaffirms their beliefs while witnessing a dramatic demonstration of the powers of their religion. This reaffirmation confirms belief that the faithful can retain good health by staying true to their religious precepts.

Even though Voodoo has ceremonies which tend to be highly localized from one region to another, they provide some measure of oneness of purpose or social consensus to the participants. When all of the individuals in the ceremony have a precise knowledge regarding the intracacies of the belief system, then a cultural consensus, or oneness of understanding, can also occur. Among adherents to Voodoo, religious faith and divine intercession are believed to transcend the particulars of the human condition, including those of physical or emotional illness. By using the services of the *houngan*, the priest in the Voodoo religion, the participants strongly feel that the *loa*, which are African spirit-dieties that have maintained their identities throughout the generations and across hemispheres, have the capabilitiy to intervene on behalf of humans and to lessen or eliminate a person's suffering and discomfort.

A number of rather striking similarities exist both in the development and the practice of Santeria and Voodoo. Like Haiti, Cuba was a receiving point for many thousands of African slaves. It was the Yoruba though, rather than the Dahomeans, who dominated the religious practices of these Afro-Cubans. As the Spanish, who controlled the island, attempted to Christianize the African slaves, they simultaneously became interested in the traditional Yoruban religious practices. After observing the rituals and learning the practices of the African priests, the Spanish implicitly sanctioned the maintenance of the traditional religion and renamed it *Santeria*, which means the worship of saints. (Gonzalez-Wippler, 1982).

This acknowledgement came about, in large part, because

these transplanted Africans, like their counterparts in Haiti, had managed to establish a parallel identification of their own gods with the saints of the Catholic religion. In this merger of the two faiths, however, the Yoruban beliefs and gods maintained their original significance so that even though Santeria represents an amalgamation of the two belief systems, the dominant aspect of the religion is clearly and distinctly African. The names of the deities and the rituals performed by the adherents are still basically the same as those that were initially introduced by the African slaves upon their arrival in Cuba in the sixteenth century. The major change that has occurred is that in Santeria, the Catholic saints have become the embodiment of the Yoruba gods. The outlook that the religion's followers have about life, including their perspectives on health and health care, is directly influenced by their faith. Further, the practice of Santaria is not confined to the ignorant and the uneducated (Gonzalez-Wippler, 1973), but encompasses persons from all social, economic and educational backgrounds.

Traditional Healing in Haiti

In Haitian society, as in most others, a person who becomes ill first attempts to treat him/herself. For minor problems, this approach is often effective because of the widespread knowledge of herbalism that exists in the country. Frequently, the individual suffering discomfort will be knowledgeable about what particular plant is effective as a treatment or cure for a certain malady, and will ingest or apply the antidote accordingly. The knowledge of such remedies is passed down from generation to generation, so there is much less trial and error involved than one might suppose.

Voodoo is practiced by most Haitian peasants, and when an illness is contracted that cannot be treated by the patient him/herself, the usual next step is a visit to a houngan. The houngan first decides whether the illness is physical or supernatural, which determines the appropriate method of treatment. For a physical infirmity, the houngan will almost certainly make use of a herbal remedy, for his knowledge of effective treatment methods in this realm extends far beyond that of the average person in the society. The nature of the service provided determines the fee that the houngan charges his client.

Haitian peasants prefer being treated by a houngan rather than a physician, for the relationship in the former case is based on trust and understanding. They trust the houngan not only for religious reasons, but as a human being, whom they have known all their lives. They have observed him under all sort of conditions, hence his personality and character are familiar and predictable. As a result, these "folk healers continue to enjoy a large clientele." (LaGuerre, 1987:47). The need for trust is, of course, so vital in a doctor-patient relationship that the formally trained physician is at a marked disadvantage, because he/she is treated suspiciously when the Haitian peasant does seek modern medical treatment. The familiarity of the houngan is a factor in inducing the trust of his client; while the unfamiliarity with the physician is, from the peasant's perspective, almost certain to generate feelings of anxiety and distrust. The situation simply represents the tendency to choose a known quantity over one that is unknown.

Since most Haitian peasants are poor, they usually visit free clinics to receive modern medical care. Regardless of the altruistic concept on which free treatment is based, the peasant is suspicious of anything free, since hard work is part of his/her mode of existence. Consequently, the absence of an even exchange relationship between doctors and patients, by the establishment of free clinics, reduces the potential utilization of health care services.

Ostensibly, the resistance to free modern medical care could be overcome through the institution of a fairly simple procedure—charging for services rendered. One approach that might be used to regularize interaction between the physician and the patient is to present a bill at the conclusion of the initial visit, and to indicate that the payment is due on some specific future date. When the patient returns to render payment, a check-up could be performed and another bill presented for that service, which would also be payable at some identified date to come, and so on. Any fee charged would have to be minimal, and might even be payable in some form other than official currency. But, in understanding that a cost would be incurred for the service, and by continuing interaction with the physician, the peasant could begin to develop the trust that would make him/her less suspicious of modern medical care, while still responding to the cultural imperatives that play an important part in determining his actions.

While *Voodoo* is believed to make a positive contribution to the health care of its followers with physical problems, it is also used to cure problems in the psychological realm. When the houngan ascertains that the problem for which help is being sought is a psychosomatic one, he attempts to discover the cause of the illness, so that it can be treated and the patient's health restored. The cause of the problem might be, for example, failure to show appropriate homage to the loa, or, it could be that an inadequate amount of respect has been paid to one's deceased ancestors. Whatever the situation, the houngan takes it upon himself to identify the physical cause of the problem, thus moving it from the category of the "untreatable" back to that of "treatable." (La Guerre, 1987).

In the process of specifying what might be a possible solution, the client becomes involved in the efforts to locate or pinpoint a method of resolution to the problem. As a result of this "person-oriented therapy," (LaGuerre, 1987) the patient is immediately involved in the idea of promising action through psychosomatic projection, instead of experiencing what Deren (1953) calls the hopeless finality of absolute abstract despair.

Thus in the interaction between the houngan and the peasant, a way is found for the patient to share in the diagnosis and to administer the solution to the problem, thus leaving that person with a much greater conception of control over his or her own life than would be gained through a more scientifically based mode of treatment. This tradition mitigates against the acceptance and use of modern health care services in which the diagnosis and treatment methods are controlled by the practitioner, and the patient plays a passive role that is limited to the application or ingestion of the prescribed remedy. Both the adjustment and adaptability functions of the Haitian peasant are greatly increased by his/her belief in Voodoo and by the acceptance of its physical and psychological means of helping to cope with difficulties as they arise.

Traditional Healing in Cuba

In Santeria, the *santero*, or practitioner, presents offerings to attract the gods, or *orishas*, so that favors can be asked of them and praises paid to them. The santero is, of course, a knowledgeable herbalist, and it is common for non-practioners of Santeria to come to one of them seeking relief from various kinds of problems. In most cases, the santero will be able to treat the difficulty with the use of a plant or herb that has curative properties of a certain medicinal nature.

Similarily well versed as the santero in the art of herbal healing, is the *babalawo*, the highest level priest in Santeria; he is the undisputed master of herbal medical treatment. He treats various kinds of illnesses and problem situations and, like the houngan in Voodoo, has a much better rapport with the common people than a trained physician is likely to develop. In addition to his expertise in areas that have physically related significance, the babalawo's advise and counsel is often sought on matters that deal with emotional and personal considerations, and he prescribes appropriate treatment for those matters as well. As a healer, the babalawo has the full confidence of the patient, because the santero believes that "they can control and rearrange all the natural phenomena around them. They believe they can effect changes in any

facet of human experience just in invoking the proper god."
(Gonzalez-Wippler, 1973:60)

For example, a healing method commonly used in Santeria,
especially when a young child needs assistance, is known as
santiguo, which means to bless. In some cases, the body of
the patient is blessed, but with special concentration given to
the area of abdomen or solar plexus. In the case of a chronic or
intestinal disease, santiguo is used as a cure, but in such
situation, the victim's stomach is also rubbed with olive oil in a
technique called a sebo de flandes. This is a special flexing of
the fingers, which are then pressed deeply into the stomach
area and brought down into the lower intestine. The santero
also lights a candle to Saint Luis Beltran, and the treatment is
stopped every few minutes to bless the stomach and to say a
prayer to the saint. This treatment often brings recovery in a
few days.

It is important for health care planners to remember that
traditional treatments with Santeria, and Voodoo present perspectives on life that include a relationship to the environment and the cosmos as integral components to the
maintenance of a healthy mind and body. They are systems
based on traditional beliefs and symbols. In conjunction with
modern health care they can work effectively and appropri-
ately for those who accept them. As such, Santeria makes
frequent use of spells, not just in matters related to health,
but as an attempt to master the various forces and con-
tingencies that anyone may face as a part of everyday life. The
spells can be used to impact a variety of situations, from
driving away bad luck to winning the favor of someone special.
In every spell, something from nature is required, whether it
be an herb, a flower, a fruit or an animal. The continuity
between human life and nature is reinforced by the santero's
belief that everything that is necessary to preserve health and
to defend against evil is available in the woods.

Clearly, traditional healing is attractive for believers in Santeria and Voodoo who distrust modern public health care, and

find it too expensive, inconvenient and impersonal. (Simpson, 1978). The degree to which indigenous people in Haiti and Cuba respond to modern health care facilities is predicated, in large part, on the manner in which these delivery systems recognize and incorporate the significant elements of their culture. The locus of their beliefs must be respected, not castigated, by the planners and staff professionals of these centers. This was rightly contended by Shils (1961) who felt that central value systems rest on human needs to be incorporated

> into something which transcends and transfigures their concrete individual existence. They have need to be in contact with symbols of an order which is larger in its dimensions than their own bodies and more central in the "ultimate" structure of reality than is their routine everyday life.

Connaissance

To fully understand the healing aspects of Voodoo, it is necessary to comprehend the concept of *connaissance*, which is the knowledge of healing and helping. The houngan gains connaissance from going through an intense study of spiritual forces and, as a result of this study, gaining an understanding of how they can be channelled to achieve the best possible end. The necessary training is a stringent process which includes several steps of elevation and tests to move from one level of knowledgeability to the next. It is the houngan's mastery of the connaissance, a mastery that is gained through diligent observation and study over a period of years that enables him to provide both remedies and insights to those who are in need of assistance. Barrett (1974) comments that the houngans are not just priests, but seers, healers, and fortune-tellers as well. They carry on the African tradition and conduct ceremonies according to a set of practices that have been handed down to them by their forefathers. Their training includes herbal medicine, psychoanalysis, music and ritual instruction, so they are well prepared to serve their clients.

It would be advantageous to integrate these traditional healers into the modern health care system because they have the trust of the peasants and they share cultural outlooks and perspectives. One approach to bringing about this integration might be to recognize the stature of the houngan within the community and to acknowledge his capacity at treating minor ailments. Thus, he could be paid a small retainer to become an *"affiliate"*, or in other words a quasi-employee of the modern health care system. As such, the houngan could also receive a referral fee for each patient that he recognizes has a malady beyond his capacity to treat and that he sends to be cared for in the modern facilities. With this referral system and the fee-for-services approach that was suggested earlier, it is possible that a much larger portion of the Haitian peasantry can be enticed into using modern health care services. There are two reasons why the houngan might be amenable to such an arrangement, aside from the money. First, he does not want his customers, who are also his friends and neighbors to suffer serious illness or death due to an infirmity that he is unable to heal. Second, despite his training, the houngan is sometimes bypassed for the *bocor*, a practitioner of magic.

A bocor is not a priest but is someone who controls and/or communicates with certain spirits and who usually uses these powers in a destructive or antagonistic fashion. These evil spirits, called baka, can be used to cause harm to people through a malevolent form of possession. It is the bocor and his practice of "black magic" that has incorrectly been portrayed as the essence of, if not the totality of Voodoo. Voodoo, according to Herskovits, (1937:153)

> "is neither the practice of black magic, nor the unorganized pathological hysteria it is so often represented to be. The gods are known to their worshipers, and the duties owed them are equally well-understood. The reward for the performance of these duties is good health, good harvests, and the goodwill of fellow men."

Likewise, Metraux writes concerning those who practice Voodoo: "Its devotees ask of it what men have always asked of religion: remedy for ills, satisfaction for needs and the hope of survival." (1959:15)

Concern for health then, and methods to maintain it are an intrinsic part of Voodoo. Acknowledging this fundamental aspect of Voodoo, rather than accepting the caricature that is so often presented in various books and television melo-dramas will lead planners of modern health care systems to think of ways in which the services offered in such facilities complement the indigenous religious practices, rather than contradict them (Barrett, 1974).

Considerations in Health Care Planning

Those persons who are involved in developing modern health care systems for use in developing countries can look to Haiti and Cuba as examples of situations where traditional patterns of belief are significant factors in designing appropri-ate treatment methods for the indigenous population. "Inter-woven among the strands making up the health of a people are the culturally related attitudes toward health itself, and to-ward the means of promoting health." (French, 1974:3)

Recognizing the role of the traditional practitioner and integrating that person into the modern health care system seems critical if the delivery of services is to reach the op-timum number of clients. Able-Smith and Leiserson (1978:102) acknowledge that "traditional medical practitioners are still widely consulted in many developing countries . . . the service provided by the traditional practitioner cannot be disregarded." It is not uncommon for a patient to consult the organized services only when treatment from the traditional practitioner has been unsuccessful. Under some circum-stances, a patient may be treated by both modern scientific and traditional practitioners at the same time. Consequently, the health planners acknowledgement of the status of the traditional practitioner within the local community, recognition that health advice or treatment from traditional practitioners may be more readily accepted than from organized services, training of natural practitioners in some modern medical practices to avoid treatments that are clearly unfavorable to health, and paying a modest salary for treatment and referral services are steps that can be taken that are in accord with the prevailing cultural imperatives. (Abel-Smith and Leiserson, 1978:102–3)

Conclusions

The prevalence of Voodoo and Santeria amongst the poor in Haiti and Cuba show that modern Western health care delivery here may be under utilized, unless it incorporates traditional perspectives into its planning. King (1965:191) posits that "a greater knowledge of the prevailing concepts and practices of folk medicine could contribute to the over-all effectiveness of a health program." As much as Westerners are inclined to use a formula approach that reflects their western cultural values rather than those of the native population, the substantial differences in national situations mean that appropriate health policy for a particular territory cannot be based on what may appear to be simple, internationally valid prescriptions (Cumper, 1984). The modes of thought and action in both countries, Haiti and Cuba, regarding illness and health are the result of African based beliefs that the people regard to have been generally effective in meeting their needs and concern. This medical heritage, despite its lack of conformity to scientific practices and procedures, continues to be a crucial element of the cultural system. Because culture is fluid, rather than static, a modern approach to health care and treatment can be developed in situations such as these, but the process must be a gradual, transitional one that respects the outlooks and perspectives of the indigenous peoples. LaGuerre (1987:88) notes that "instead of perpetuating the arrogance of Western Medicine, the ability of the health professional to adapt to local culture is of utmost importance."

Bibliography

Abel-Smith, Brian and Alcira Leiserson (1978) Poverty, Development and Health Policy. Geneva: World Health Organization

Barrett, Leonard (1974) Soul Force. Garden City, N.Y.: Anchor Books.

Bastide, Roger (1971) African Civilizationns in the New World. New York: Harper & Row, 1971

Bourguignon, Erika (1970) Ritual Dissociation and Possession Belief in Caribbean Negro Religion. Pp. 87–102 in Norman Whitten and John Szwed (eds.), Afro-American Anthropology. New York: Free Press.

Courlander, Harold and Remy Bastien (1966) Religion and Politics in Haiti. Washington, D.C.: Institute for Cross Cultural Research.

Cumper, G. E. (1984) Determinants of Health Levels in Developing Countries. Letchworth, England: Research Studies Press, Ltd.

Deren, Maya (1953) Divine Horsemen: The Voodoo Gods of Haiti. London: Thames and Hudson.

French, Ruth (1974) The Dynamics of Health Care. New York: McGraw-Hill, 1974.

Gonzalez-Wippler, Migene (1973) Santeria: African Magic in Latin America. New York: The Julian Press.

Gonzalez-Wippler, Migene (1982) The Santeria Experience. Englewood Cliffs, N.J.: Prentice-Hall.

Haskins, Jim (1978) Voodoo and Hoodoo, New York: Stein and Day.

Herskovits, Melville (1937) Life in a Haitian Valley. New York: Alfred Knopf Co.

Herskovits, Melville (1958) The Myth of the Negro Past. Boston: Beacon Press

King, Robert L. (1965) Health Facilities Construction in the Caribbean. Pp. 176–90 in A. Curtis Wilgus (ed.), The Caribbean: Its Health Problems. Gainesville, Fla.: University of Florida Press.

LaGuerre, Michel (1987) Afro-Caribbean Folk Medicine South Hadley, Mass. Bergin and Garvey publishers

Metraux, Albert (1959) Voodoo in Haiti. Oxford: Oxford University Press.

Price-Mars, Heab (1928) Ainsi Parla L'Oncle. Paris: Impr. de Compiegne

Shils, Edward (1961) Centre and Periphery. Pp. 117–30 in the Logic of Personal Knowledge. Glencove, Ill.: Free Press.

Simpson, George (1978) Black Religions in the New World. New York: Columbia University Press.

Whiting John, and Irving Child (1953) Child Training and Personality. New Haven: Yale University Press.

CHAPTER 9

Coyote Returns: Integration of American Indian Indigenous Practitioners in Mental Health Programs

William Willard and Robin A. LaDue

The integration of traditional American healers is advocated. The U.S. Indian Health Service sanctions such integration in its national policy, encouraging a holistic approach to health care. Resistance comes from both, modern as well as traditional practitioners. Indigenous healers see such integration as a threat to their cultural healing practices and fear of having to take a subordinate role to modern medical professionals. Integration of traditional providers into modern health care delivery systems has greater acceptance in mental health services than in physical medicine.

Introduction

THE USE OF NATURAL HELPERS AND TRADITIONAL HEALERS in American Indian health programs has been advocated by Indian communities, tribal governments, the National Indian Health Board and the Indian Health Service (IHS). The IHS,

115

Office of Mental Health Programs, operates under a national policy which reflects a holistic approach to health care, and an attitude of respect for the place held by traditional healing practices in contemporary Indian life. (For complete IHS policy statement, see Appendix A.)

However, the actual formal linkage between traditional healers, and the modern health care establishment has occurred in only a few, isolated cases.

The policy of sanctioning the involvement of traditional healing practices in a holistic approach to mental health appears to be one of great potential in extending the access of treatment for people who might otherwise have restricted, non-existent, or inappropriate therapeutic facilities. During this time of budget cutbacks and decreasing services, such a policy *b* its implementation become even more important. Although the integration of informal helping systems has not been explored to any depth, in some geographic areas the concept has been documented.

Ruiz and Langrod (1976) in a New York City out-patient mental health center found that many of their patients were also visiting mediums and spiritual healers. The authors then sought to develop a liaison program to bring the two systems together. The plan included hiring mediums as community mental health workers and developing a pre-service training program for the staff for familiarization with the approaches to the medium and spiritualists.

Ramesh and Hyma (1981) reported a stand-off situation in which indigenous medical practitioners in an Indian city, express reluctance to cooperate in becoming integrated. The practitioners felt that integration could threaten their individual cultural healing characteristics and force them into a dependent subordinate role to scientific medicine. Dual systems they felt preserved independent cultural medical systems. The resistance of practitioners of any medical system toward incorporation into any other should therefore be taken into account in the implementation of any system's coordination, particularly in cases where there have been long-time histories of mistrust between the proponents and practitioners of the two systems.

There are some circumstances in which traditional healers are positive about official recognition. In Kenya, Katz and Kimani (1982) found that traditional medicine is a viable and frequently used option for an urban population with ready access to cosmopolitan medicine. There are modification in practice imposed by the urban environment and modifications in the types of patients and conditions seen resulting from the patients' choice of options. A new role is gradually evolving for the traditional medical practitioner, one which is complementary to that of the cosmopolitan physician. Traditional practitioners are eager to be officially recognized and can be a valuable resource in providing health care. This is particularly true in the city where they tend to be full-time, with their clinics located in the center of the residential areas.

The slight available literature on the operational functioning of mental health programs for American Indians which do take a holistic approach including traditional healing practices, led to the launching of a survey project in July, 1981. The survey was intended to determine the current state of integration of traditional and non-traditional folk medicine practitioners into mental health services programs for American Indians. A review of the literature on integration of indigenous traditional and modern medical practitioners into national health programs indicates that there appears to be a greater acceptance of indigenous practitioners in mental health services than in physical medicine, and equally important, an acceptance by indigenous practitioners of roles in mental health services (Araneta, 1977).

In the United States, mental health services to American Indians are provided through: 1) the Indian Health Service, Office of Mental Health programs, which is part of the U.S. Public Health Service. Eligibility for the services of the Indian Health Service is limited to people who are officially enrolled members of federally recognized groups with reservation land bases held in federal trusteeship. Access to health services is redefined by federal policy from time to time, but is frequently limited to persons living on or near reservations, who also qualify under all other eligibility rules; 2) tribal health programs located on or near reservation communities. Access to services is usually limited to enrolled members of the particular tribe recognized as the corporate governing and land holding body of the particular reservation; 3) state and local government funded mental health programs with eligibility for services determined by particular program regulations and almost never restricted to an American Indian population; and 4) Alaskan native corporation mental health programs which provide services to corporation members.

Methodology

The survey was sent to mental health programs serving American Indian populations in the United States and Canada. Agency names were acquired in a variety of ways, i.e. tribal agencies, IHS, word-of-mouth, and personal knowledge. The actual survey process had three phases: 1) a general letter of inquiry; 2) a follow-up letter focusing on program and population specifics; and 3) site visit whenever and wherever possible.

The first inquiry letter asked if the recipient could identify any American Indian mental health service programs which integrate (or link) with either traditional or non-traditional healers. If an affirmative response was received, the respondent was sent a second inquiry letter asking the following:

1. Is the folk practitioner an official member of the health services program?
2. Is the practitioner a paid member of the program?
3. Is there a cross referral arrangement?
4. Is there a referral arrangement?
5. Are there training sessions involving folk practitioners and all other members of the health service?

6. Are there training sessions involving practitioners and health service members?
7. Is there an official policy concerning involvement of folk practitioners in health services?

Findings

Replies to the survey have generally been that there is no involvement with either traditional or non-traditional indigenous healers, as indicated by the following replies:

> "We tried working with traditional healers, and had some interference from some of the more Christian members of our community and the program was terminated." U.S.A., Kansas

> "Formal linkages have never been established because staff feels that to do so would diminish the power that healers have or 'take away' from the process." U.S.A., Arizona

> "The implication is that traditional approaches to healing must always remain in their purest form and not become a part of the modern behavioral health treatment setting." U.S.A., Arizona

> "Our position has been that traditional healing is a private family and community matter which should be encouraged without a formal linkage on our part." U.S.A., New Mexico

A reply which was particularly intriguing was one in which a non-Indian psychologist wrote that he is not supposed to know about any indigenous curers in his geographic area. A telephone call brought out the meaning behind the seemingly cryptic written reply. The local Native American communities simply did not want the identities of their curers to be known to non-Indians. Therefore, the psychologist respondent "is not supposed to know" about the local healers.

Other further personal inquiry found that some Native American religions do not regard the official mental health professionals and programs as being effective therapies for Native Americans. Rather, it is held that only the practitioners sanctioned by these religions and their respective communities are regarded as effective therapists for Native Americans.

Survey respondents who indicated an involvement with either traditional or non-traditional practitioners gave a less wide range of replies:

> "What we are promoting is an understanding of the importance of the traditional healer in the cross-cultural orientation of our own health workers." Saskatchewan, Canada

> "We have been able to gradually put together a full comprehensive community mental health program which is by design, culturally relevant throughout. Traditional healers are a most important—if not crucial—component of our program." Idaho, U.S.A.

In the United States, the Indian Health Service (IHS) has in informal policy of allowing local I.H.S. Service Unit decisions on recognition, level of involvement; and fee for service allowance for either traditional or non-traditional healers.

Therefore, there is a positive answer to Foster's question: "To ask about the possible use of traditional healers in national health services is to ask an incomplete partial question. The real question, is, should any or all forms of alternative health care systems and their practitioners be recognized as legitimate and efforts be made to incorporate them into government health services?" (Foster, 1978; 261.)

In allowing for local option, then there is no conflict with national policy on the basis of exclusion of any particular healing tradition. Analysis of the survey data brought out elements not immediately seen with respect to the question, whether or not to integrate indigenous healers into modern health care delivery systems.

It was found that in some areas there were no American Indian curers. Available were only the official mental health services, and acculturation had erased any former native healing tradition. Official mental health services personnel often had no knowledge of any native system, be it traditional or non-traditional. There may have been several active practitioners with many clients in the particular area, but such knowledge was not passed on to mental health officials.

In some mental health centers a favored few traditional healers were brought in to give lectures and demonstrations to clinic staff during staff training sessions. However, these individuals were not well screened. They may or may not have been respected curers of a native traditional healing system. Actually, some mental health professionals had accepted an individual as the official native healer who, in fact was only a marginal individual, skilled only in how to be acceptable to the psychiatrists and social workers. The reason for this is that native healing systems maintain an aloof attitude toward involvement with any other healing system.

Discussion

Araneta, 1977 questions the benefits of a collaboration between modern and traditional mental health professionals. His objections are twofold:

> "First, does collaboration with indigenous healers provide significantly better therapeutic results in dealing with psychiatric impairment in minority groups and subcultures? And second, does collaboration with indigenous healers inevitably foster the perpetuation of animistic, magical, supra- and preter-naturally oriented cultural patterns that have limited capacity to incorporate technological and social progress, resulting in their being delegated to the role of a colonialized minority?" (Araneta: 1977:73).

The answer to the first point Araneta makes, on the basis of our survey is that flexibility in mental health programs is an essential factor. If local cultures are ignored or worse, suppressed by a monolithic national health policy, mental health problems for national minority groups may simply be exacerbated without the opportunity for either category of therapy.

Araneta's second point does not recognize that the cultural patterns which he suggests, will limit the cultural incorporation of technological and social progress, and are as descriptive of any cultural group, majority or minority, colonizing or colonized. In our survey, we do not find that psychiatrists and other mental health professionals are available on a daily basis in any Native American community in either the United States or Canada and certainly not elsewhere in the Americas.

It is recommended therefore that national health policies are flexible, because indigenous healing systems often persist as separate entities, and a fair percentage of indigenous curers will accept integration into other systems. In contrast, many modern health care professionals resist involvement of indigenous practitioners. Likewise, traditional religious groups do not accept practitioners identified with other religions as part of official health services, nor permit involvement in modern mental health services by their own curers. A large number of American Indian communities do not now have practitioners from any healing tradition other than modern mental health professionals, such as psychiatrists, psychologists and social workers of Euro-American official tradition who, as noted, may not be readily accessible.

The question of what *"tradition"* is involved, has received a variety of replies reflecting our current social and cultural environment. Indigenous healing practices derived from the historic cultural traditions are apparently not involved in any direct way with modern mental health programs. In the Southwest where there has been much ethnographic description of native medical systems, there seems to be a major cultural change under way with some strongly resurgent healing traditions with historic cultural roots.

What is meant by traditional Indian medicine is found by the survey, to vary from one community to another in important ways not necessarily reflecting the historic native cultures. Christian denominations and Christian derived denominations, are traditional Indian religions in many communities. There is a general replacement of native practices by

Christianity throughout the United States, which include curing and beliefs about health and illness. Locally, the church of Jesus Christ of Latter Day Saints has become influential through its Lamanite Mission activity. The Native American Church has been actively evangelizing since the later 1890's in the U.S. Plains States, Canadian Prairie Provinces, the U.S. Southwest, and in other areas of the U.S. and Canada as well. In the Northwest, the Indian Shaker Church is active in many Native American communities.

There are also local churches organized around the personal visions of Christianity of some local leaders, without affiliations beyond one particular community. Fundamentalist Christian denominations have been established in many, if not all, Native American communities in the United States. These churches have a strong emphasis on supernatural healing based on New Testament examples.

In the United States, a contemporary Shamanism seems to have been developing through the 1970's and is now considered by people in several areas of the United States to be *"Indian Medicine"* and to be practiced by *"Medicine Persons."* Initially, the syncretic nature of this contemporary Shamanism was puzzling because of the amalgamation of components from disparate cultural traditions. The explanation appears to be in part that in the 1970's, some American Indians had not grown up in their ancestral cultures. Consequently, they then "mixed and matched" cultural items into a new synthesis of contemporary American Indian cultures. Alongside this new synthesis, a second movement has been adding other items to the cultural mosaic.

Healers, drawing their methods from many sources, have appeared in both urban and reservation communities. These practitioners frequently utilize nothing from any American Indian culture of the past, but instead, use Tarot cards, crystal balls, Asian and European herbal remedies, science fiction literature and astrology in a very syncretic evolution. All of this seems to be part of an evolving system of supernatural therapies derived from many sources; traditional religions,

Christianity, Shamanistic healing rituals, and spiritualism, for some examples. The phenomena has been pointed out by Foster (1978) in relationship to a general worldwide trend of scientific medicine and supernatural therapies rapidly replacing all of the traditional naturalistic therapies. Foster feels the major reason for this is that the two complementary systems are simply more effective in meeting human health needs. Scientific medical therapies are sometimes unsatisfactory in the treatment of many chronic illnesses, whereas supernatural therapies sometimes have a more palliative affect for the chronically ill.

Conclusion

The concept of integrating both scientific medicine and indigenous medical traditions have been advocated. The argument for incorporation or integration is frequently based on two perspectives: first, that of economy. The number of physicians trained in scientific medicine available to Native American communities is not adequate to meet health services needs. Therefore, in order to meet the urgent need for health care, the already existing indigenous practitioner should be incorporated as rapidly as possible into the national health services system.

The second argument is that indigenous curers share in the same worldview as the patients and therefore are more acceptable and can proceed to care in ways which are culturally acceptable to all concerned. Then too, medical systems, whether scientific medicine or any other, are parts of total cultural patterns and in form and content reflect patterns and values that may not be immediately observable. Therefore, if both categories of practitioners can be involved in the same system the benefits of both curing systems can be provided for the service population in culturally relevant environments. Thus, the key topic is utilization of traditional medicine because health, illness and disease are as much social and cultural phenomena as they are biological. The health service needs of Native American communities are not likely to be met by modern health services alone.

Responses to the integration of Shamanistic practitioners in mental health programs have the potential range for rejection, assimilation, selective integration and total integration, all at the local level of community culture and society. Policies, formal or informal, are only effective as they may become operational at the service delivery level, the local community and the individual person.

Presented at the American Political Science Association Convention, New York, 1983

Appendix A

U.S. PUBLIC HEALTH SERVICE, INDIAN HEALTH SERVICE OFFICE OF MENTAL HEALTH PROGRAMS

PROPOSED POLICY AND PROCEDURES
CHAPTER 0
SECTION 0.0

TRADITIONAL INDIAN PRACTICES AND MENTAL HEALTH SERVICES

1. *Purpose:*
To set forth the policy of the Indian Health Service (IHS) to reflect: a) a holistic approach to health care; and b) an attitude of respect for the place held by traditional healing practices in contemporary Indian life.

2. *Policy:*

   A. It is the policy of the Indian Health Service Office of Mental Health Programs to view individuals as whole persons with many interdependent culturally influenced physical, social, psychological and spiritual needs. This policy also recognizes that illness may derive from, or be complicated by, any need or combination of needs improperly met or managed. Thus, the best treatment plan is one which takes into account the many needs of the person while still viewing him/her as a unitary whole.

B. The I.H.S. Office of Mental Health Programs, from its inception, has recognized the value and efficacy of traditional beliefs, ceremonies, and practices in the healing of the body, mind and spirit. Faith is most often an integral part of the healing process and provides support for purposeful living. It is, therefore, the policy of the I.H.S. Office of Mental Health Programs to encourage a climate of respect and acceptance in which an individual's private traditional beliefs may become a part of the healing and harmonizing force within her/his life.

3. *Procedures*
   1. Members of the I.H.S. Mental Health staff are encouraged, as a part of health care teams, to adopt an holistic approach to preventive and curative health.
   2. Mental Health clients, and other I.H.S. patients, shall not be discouraged from seeking out the unique benefits which are derived from native healing practices and other religious resources.
   3. When a patient requests assistance in obtaining the services of a native practitioner, he/she should not be discouraged from doing so and a native practitioner may be contacted and space or privacy may be provided within a hospital room for a ceremony. However, when payment is required for such services, the use of contract health care funds to pay for native healer consultation may be authorized only when the treating physician has certified that such consultation is medically necessary for the patient's well being and it is determined that the service is within CHS priorities.

4. Since a person's religious and native beliefs are often very personal, the patient's right to privacy must be respected in these matters. I.H.S. employees should avoid uninvited probing or interference in a patient's private beliefs. Many Indian patients prefer to say nothing about these native beliefs and practices. This is a right which must be respected.

5. In implementing this policy, I.H.S. mental health staff need to be aware of, sensitive to, and respectful of traditional beliefs and practices in the healing process.

References

Araneta, Enrique. (1977) *Traditional Healing: New Science or New Colonialism?* Philip Singer, ed. New York: Conch Magazine.

Foster, George M. (1978) *Medical Anthropology.* New York: John Wiley and Sons.

Katz, Sydney S., Katz, Selig H., and V. N. Kimani. (1982) "The Making of an Urban Mganga: New Trends in Traditional Medicine in Urban Kenya." *Medical Anthropology*, Vol. 6, Number 2: 91–112, Spring.

Kimani, Violet N. (1981) "Attempts to Coordinate the Work of the Traditional and Modern Doctors in Nairobi in 1980." *Social Science and Medicine*, 15B: 421–22.

Ramesh and Hyma, *Traditional and Modern Medical Systems.* Ray Elling, ed. (1981) *Social Science and Medicine* (Special Issue) Vol. 15A, No. 2. New York: Pergamon Press.

Ruiz, P. and Langrod, J. (1976) "The Role of Folk Healers in Community Mental Health Services." *Community Mental Health Journal*, 12(4):392–398.

Public Health and Traditional Beliefs

CHAPTER 10

Human Behavior and Health in Developing Africa

Frank L. Lambrecht

In an unchanged human environment the transmission of infectious diseases tends to stabilize in a set of patterns which, in the long run, may be beneficial to the relationship between host, parasite and eventual vector. However, human behavior, whether individual or collective, constantly modifies environmental conditions thereby altering, for better or for worse, the partnership between man, his parasites and their vectors. The large-scale development operations in tropical countries have generally intensified the endemicity and spread of parasitic diseases, especially those associated with water impoundment and irrigation schemes. The prior assessment of health hazards that could result from environmental changes caused by development operations should help planning adequate countermeasures or prevent health problems to occur altogether. Human culture and behavior play an important role in disease distribution both in spread and in restraint.

Diseases, Human Environment and Behavior

DISEASES AND MORE PARTICULARLY INFECTIOUS DISEASES, are closely linked to the ecosystem of the human host in which cultural oriented behavior plays an important role. The ecological approach—the comprehensive attention given to the mutual relations between organisms and their environment—underlines the complicity between environment and disease agents. It also focuses attention on multiple effects of human action that alter the relationship between people and their environment, often with important medical consequences.

Poor health and the high endemicity of communicable diseases are often directly or indirectly the result of socio-economic conditions. In a short article entitled: "Life seen from a medieval latrine," Moore (1981), describes the finding during the excavation for a new housing development in Worchester, England, of the lower part of a medieval barrel latrine filled with organic material. The analyses of the contents revealed seeds, pollen, vegetable debris, insects and a high concentration of eggs belonging to the human parasites, whipworm and roundworm. The presence of these intestinal parasites reflects the low standard of living conditions and want of hygiene during those times. Dunn (1968, 1972) demonstrated that the species and incidence of parasites infecting hunter-gatherers populations vary with the diversity and complexity of the ecosystem, in rural villages with population density, house types, domestic animals, subsistence strategy, mobility of the inhabitants, and other environmental variables.

In the prevention and control of communicable diseases aspects of human behavior and environment often do not receive the attention they demand. Curiously enough because the sources of infections can usually be linked to these factors. The term human behavior is not restricted to individuals but includes the activities of family groups and communities, religious practices, the aspects of nomadism, type of profession, and diet. The term environment not only concerns conditions found in the general surroundings but also those of the domestic habitat.

The relationship between human behavior, environment and parasitic diseases can be demonstrated in most cases. Under theoretical stable conditions of unchanging populations and environment, the occurrence of diseases can be expected to fall into a fixed pattern, eventually reaching a state of tolerance/equilibrium between host and parasite, possibly leading to local races. Such a situation could develop in geographically isolated populations but is very rare in our rapidly evolving societies. Indeed, never in the history of human social evolution have there been such drastic, country-wide changes as in Africa during this century. With the western colonisation of the continent the way of life of whole populations was transformed from that of stone-age societies to 20th century communities in half a century. Such a sudden and large-scale change requires profound social and biological adjustments.

The impact of western civilization during the first decades of the colonial period may have been insignificant due to the sparse European occupation and the lack of communications. The sudden change came with the rapid development of road systems and modern transportation, including aviation, just before World War II and especially after the war when substantial loan funds were poured into the previous colonies, now called developing countries of the third world.

Whereas the development of the prewar colonies was understandably slow, that of the post-colonial times was furious, impetuous and often heedless. The underlying aim of some of the development plans was sometimes political, often one-sided and frequently with complete disregard to ecological or social consequences. Many times it resulted in serious public health problems.

The construction of the Sennar dam on the Blue Nile in 1925, built to irrigate and raise crops in half a million acres in the Gezirah region of the Sudan is one of the early examples of an extensive man-made disease-promoting environment. The irrigated fields were soon invaded by fresh-water snails that are the intermediate vectors (carriers) of the liver-fluke disease (Schistosomiasis also called Bilharzia) and by anopheles mosquitoes that carry malaria. During the 1950 malaria epidemic, hundreds of people died while the number of incapacitated sick was such that a third of the crops remained unharvested (Gaitskell, 1959).

Large-scale Environmental Changes

The Gezirah and other early examples of health-related environmental changes have not always been taken as warning by later developers. Over the last two or three decades we are witnessing a dramatic increase in human exposure to diseases as a result of large-scale agricultural development schemes, water management projects and opening up of new lands for settlement and exploitation.

The rapid increase of malaria and bilharzia in the wake of dam-building clearly proves the health-linked hazards. Six major dams have been built in Africa alone in the last twenty years. Hundreds of miles of swift-running water courses have been transformed into thousands of hectares of lake surfaces and vast areas of irrigated land. The increase of disease vectors requiring an aquatic environment for breeding, such as snails and mosquitoes, has been consumerate with this expanse of surface waters.

It is not so much the extension of water surface, from stream into a large lake, that accounts for the increase of mosquito breeding—few larvae will be found beyond the first ten meters from the shore—than well the lengthening of the shoreline itself. The damming of the Upper Volta River transformed 400 Km. of river (= 800 Km. riverbanks) into Volta Lake of approximately 8500 Km2—the largest man-made lake in the world with a shoreline estimated at about 6400 Km. The transformation of 800 Km. original river bank into 6400 Km. shoreline provides, therefore, eight times more potential mosquito breeding places.

Not only will the transformation of a river into a lake affect mosquito breeding quantitatively, that is the amount of breeding potential, but also qualitatively, that is the increase of choice of ecological niches and chances of species diversity. The waters of the lake, following the contour-lines of its basin, will form creeks, back-waters, seepage areas and swamps that greatly diversify mosquito larvae habitats, enhanced by subsequent development of grasses, reeds, shrubs and other water-edge vegetation. The growth of floating water-plants encourages the establishment of mosquitoes. The same processes also favors the invasion of vector-snails which in the protected creaks of the lake shore find ideal conditions for proliferation. The extensive irrigation network, often an integral part of water management, is responsible for extending numerous vector habitats far beyond the range of the original water course. Introduced in an arid environment, irrigation systems promote the establishment of water-borne vectors and pathogens previously absent from the area.

Whereas environmental changes induced by development projects could be directly responsible for changes in communicable disease patterns, endemicity and incidence, indirectly related factors also greatly affect the well-being of populations: migration, relocation, transit camps, occupation of virgin land, replacement of natural vegetation by crops, and road-building.

The trauma, psychological as well as physiological, of the Gwembe Tonga people displaced by the rising waters of Lake Kariba after the construction of the dam on the Zambezie River in Zimbabwe, was the subject of a detailed study of Tayer Scudder (1966, 1972).

The magnitude of the problem associated with the relocation of populations after the formation of an artificial lake and the flooding of their homeland can be judged from the number of people involved: Aswan: 100,000; Kainji: 42,000; Kariba: 56,000; Kossou: 80,000; Volta: 70,000. Health hazards related to the construction of dams also include the labor force and satellite activities. For instance, the building of the Kainji dam in Nigeria, by far not the most important of dams constructed in West Africa, involved more than 20,000 professional men for over four years. Health problems and accidents were enhanced by overcrowding, poor housing and sanitation. Besides the labor force, hundreds of traders and other people flocked to the area seeking their fortune and for whom no housing nor adequate sanitation was prepared. As a result, various infectious diseases became rampant (Obeng, 1969).

The development of new areas invariably includes new access roads with the establishment of villages and trading centers. These act as stepping stones for the propagation of vectors and diseases into the newly opened regions. The construction of roads in itself is often instrumental to the spread of disease vectors breeding in burrow pits, ditches and culverts during the rains, especially mosquitoes, while also providing favorable snail habitats (Lambrecht, 1981).

In inhabited areas, breeding sites of mosquitoes are mostly man-made. In a village in eastcentral Nigeria, the main source of mosquito breeding occurred in water stored in clay pots. Family compounds carried on an average eighty water-pots. Over a one-year period of observation, 36 percent of these contained larvae of 14 mosquito species, including three potential yellow fever carriers (Peterson & Lambrecht, 1976).

Recognizing the association between the transmission of diseases and primitive water supply methods, the World Health Organization is giving great attention, and is sponsoring a number of projects, to provide safe piped-water systems to urban and rural towns and villages. Besides the reduction of mosquito breeding, public water systems will help decrease contact between schistosoma-infected streams and villagers who are forced to bathe and draw water at these places. It will help prevent infections with Dracunculiasis (Guinea worm) from contaminated wells, and minimize risks of contracting sleeping sickness in places where water has to be drawn from tsetse fly infested rivers. The provision of safe piped water would also avoid hazards of water-borne typhoid fevers, cholera, amoebiasis, and various other infections.

Diseases Associated with the Raising of Certain Crops

Besides possible contact with zoonotic diseases when people transpose virgin land into agricultural fields, certain types of crops could, intrinsically, become a factor in promoting and sustaining infectious diseases.

Flooded rice fields cause multiple health problems. Firstly, mosquitoes and snails breeding will occur over large areas with risks of transmission of the parasites they carry. Secondly, as the rice plants grow, the increasing shade at various stages provides a choice of habitats for different species of mosquitoes and snails. Diversity is enhanced when fields are not properly weeded and other plants further increase habitat types. Thirdly, breeding and transmission occurs throughout the year in regions where two rice crops are won per year. Furthermore, short periods during which rice fields are drying up are usually not sufficient to eliminate the vector populations as several species of snails are known to withstand dryness through aestivation, as do the eggs of some mosquito species.

Flooded rice plantations have contributed notoriously to the spread of bilharzia. In Africa, the Middle East, parts of South America and the Caribbean, bilharzia is caused by the man-to-man transmitted *Schistosoma mansoni* and *Schistosoma haematobium* carried by various genera of freshwater snails. In the Far East, however, where the disease is caused by *Schistosoma japonicum*, the parasite is also found in various animal hosts, including the water buffalo. Through its close association with man during the preparation of the rice fields, the water buffalo is of great epidemiological significance in maintaining and spreading the disease.

Ripening rice will attract field rodents and other small mammals some of which are carriers of leptospirosis (Weil's disease). From the urine of infected animals the parasite gains access and infects rice cultivators standing bare-legged in contaminated water.

On a smaller scale but possibly more widespread is the mosquito breeding potential in "axil-leave plants" where rain- or dew-water collects in the cavity formed at the junction of the U-shaped leaf with the stem. This type of larvae habitat is found in banana trees, cocoyam, pineapple, and various plants used for making hedges. A one-year study in Nigeria showed the presence in the four kinds of plants mentioned of twelve mosquito species, including three potential yellow fever vectors (Peterson & Lambrecht, 1976).

Some seven hundred species of Bamboo grow profusely in many regions of the world, in low- and highlands. Common to all varieties is the hollow stem composed of partitioned nodes. When the stem is cut, the exposed part of a node forms a hollow cup which when filled with rain-water provides an ideal larval habitat, especially favored by the yellow fever mosquito. In many regions of Africa, bamboo groves are grown at the periphery of villages because of the plant's many uses. Used as guide-poles in the cultivation of yams, the staple food in West Africa, the bamboo stems offer mosquito breeding sites over large areas of cultivated land; used for fencing, mosquito breeding is brought unawaringly to home and gardens. Grain crops attract and promote the multiplication of rodents that are potential carriers of disease agents such as leptospirosis, plague, typhus, and various virus diseases. Rat-bites may cause infections. The traditional storage of grain in primitive vessels and bins is an additional threat of bringing diseases close to living quarters. The plantation of trees for windbreaks, soil stabilization, erosion prevention, firewood reserve, also may incur some health risks. Generally, large forests in arid areas will change climate and environment that could favour the invasion of certain insects and animals, and their parasites. A recent study in the Lambwe Valley of Western Kenya showed the invasion by flies of a pine-tree plantation thereby extending the flybelt, previously confined to the valley, far upon the previously fly-free slopelands. It was especially *L. camara*, a plant introduced from South America as an ornamental shrub, that provided opportunity to the fly to spread into peridomestic habitats, resulting in a severe sleeping sickness outbreak during the years 1963–66 in the Alego District.

Man-made Disease Environments

The transmission of relapsing fever in East Africa, a disease carried by ticks, relies on a close contact cycle between parasite, vector and host that, regionally, may include the domestic pig. The contact is conditioned by the convergence of contributing factors, including: type of house plan, location of sleeping quarters and type of bed, presence and kind of domestic animals kept inside the dwelling, presentness of permanent wood-fire. Relapsing fever is an example of a "stabilized" host-parasite-vector association. People who have been exposed to local strains, such as found in East Africa, acquire a partial immunity that is not permanent and does not protect them from infections of strains in the lowlands. It is said that when inhabitants from endemic relapsing fever areas leave for other places, to seek work, to visit or as prisoners, they take with them a small box with infected ticks which they feed on themselves occasionally in order to keep their immunity until they return home and are once more exposed to the "natural" transmission cycle.

Insects and other animal pests are often associated and depend upon certain types of human dwellings and the materials used in their construction. Unhygienic houses, prevalent in most of the tropical underdeveloped countries, are conducive to the circulation of parasitic infections. Cracked mud-walls offer hiding places for numerous insect vectors: bedbugs (typhus), reduviid bugs (Chagas' disease), ticks (rickettsioses, relapsing fever), mosquitoes (malaria, filariases, viruses), cockroaches and other crawling insects that may contaminate food with bacteria and other disease agents. Primitive dwellings provide shelter and close contact with various "domestic" animal pests such as rats which carry diseases. On a larger scale, the unplanned, unorganized and often unlawful "shanty towns" that grow at the periphery of most tropical cities are major sources of epidemics started by the influx of disease-carrying newcomers and fostered by conditions favoring the proliferation of disease vectors. Moreover, many squatters

refrain from seeking medical help at the government dispensary or hospital afraid to disclose their illegal immigration
status.

Health-related Environmental Changes Due to Natural Causes

During the late 1960's, irregular but sudden increases in
cases of human sleeping sickness in the Okavango Swamp
region puzzled and worried the Botswana's health authorities.
The cause(s) of these upflares was studied by a team of the
World Health Organization in 1966–68. The investigations
indicated that, first of all, the expansion of irrigated fields
along the "molapos" (seasonal rivers), while greatly extending
the growing season and capacity of crops in the 9-months dry
country, increased the exposure of the farmers to the tsetse
flies inhabiting the molapo vegetation, and the risks of contracting sleeping sickness. But other events that contributed
to the risks were found to have a natural cause. A study of the
history of sleeping sickness cases on the western fringes of the
swamps revealed a series of events that seemed to correlate
with variations in the flood-waters of the Okavango River and
the Okavango Swamps, its inland delta. It should be explained here that human sleeping sickness in Botswana is of
the acute type, a disease carried and maintained in several
species of wild animals. The interplay of seasonal migration of
animal reservoirs and variations in the extent of human occupation of the flood plains caused by fluctuating flood cycles
in some years could explain differences in the degree of
human contact with tsetse flies and carrier-animals that, likewise, respond to these fluctuations, as seen in figure 1
(Lambrecht, 1972).

Social and Cultural Aspects of Epidemiology

Epidemiology studies the selective distribution of diseases
and their meaning. Investigations concern populations and

Figure 1
Variations in the extent of flooding of the Okavango River, Botswana

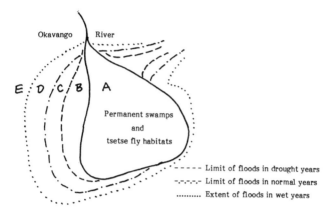

.... Extent of floods in wet years

A. About 5,000 square miles of permanent swamps with scattered permanent tsetse fly habitats: continuous risks of sleeping sickness transmission to swamp-dwelling populations, occasional travellers and hunters.

B. High degree of exposure to sleeping sickness infections of floodplain cultivators when in drought years they are forced to farm closer to the tsetse fly-infested swamp areas.

C. Low degree of contact with tsetse flies during "normal" flood years when the open floodplains receive enough moisture for raising crops with only scant fly contact.

D. During exceptionally high floods: increasing degree of man-fly contact when tsetse and potential animal reservoirs of human sleeping sickness, especially the "efficient" carrier *Redunca redunca* (reedbuck), are driven by the flood waters into the populated areas of surrounding country.

E. Surrounding country with human settlements and cattle. Scattered pockets of tsetse habitats in the woodland savannah outside the human settlements are only low sleeping sickness risks in normal years.

samples of populations rather than hospitalized or clinical cases. Epidemiology is both descriptive and analytic, encompassing the origin and the cause of the disease besides the pattern of distribution. Epidemiology is a powerful tool for understanding disease behavior and thereby a powerful means to its control when the study has shown its correlation to specific environmental factors. Epidemiology, therefore, has a close relation to ecology. The environment of a population and disease under study, include factors as: geography, topography and climate, population characteristics as: urban or rural, age and sex structure, diet, industries, religion, and so on.

In tropical countries where parasitic diseases are often closely associated to socio-economic and ecological conditions, factors may have a far more significant role in disease distribution than in the industrialized world where natural environmental factors have been largely eliminated or altered.

Diseases which are transmitted by an intermediate carrier (= vector), and most tropical diseases are, are entirely dependent, of course, upon the distribution of the vector which, itself, is dependent upon the environmental conditions that allow it to complete its life-cycle. It is in this respect that geography, topography, soil characteristics, vegetation types and climate play a predominant role in the distribution of vector-borne diseases. The geographical and altitudinal location of a village will or will not expose its inhabitants to certain diseases. This also goes for whether one lives in the forest, in the savannah, along a river, in wildlife areas, near swamps, on irrigated lands, in dry or wet areas, and so on.

Certain group behavior, such as cultural or religious practices, may act as a stimulus for disease transmission or a deterrent. For example: the large numbers of clay pots left in the sacred shrines in Nigeria are a constant source of mosquito breeding; flower vases on tombstones in numerous Seychelles Islands cemeteries also fulfill the role of proliferic mosquito breeding places; mosquito larvae are commonly found in the ablution bowls in toilets of muslim countries; cement footbaths in some muslim mosques have been found the foci of skin-fungus; the habit of some oriental populations of eating raw fish exposes them to infection with the Chinese liver fluke; in warm countries where the soil is often contaminated with larvae of hookworm, walking barefoot invites infections with this worm. Other customs, on the contrary, are preventive against certain infections: the habit of boiling water is a strong deterrent against a hord of parasitic diseases; the abstention of pork meat in the Jewish and Muslim religion protects the followers from infections by pork tape-worm; vegetarians avoid risks of infections by a number of parasitic worms that are risks to people eating uncontrolled, uncooked meats.

Within a population, all members may not be exposed to the same degree of disease organisms. Women and children are more exposed to bites of riverine insects that carry diseases—tsetse flies for sleeping sickness, black flies are carriers of river blindness—or to infections by schistosoma organisms in the stream or Guinea worm in a contaminated step-well. Hunting or honey-collecting by the men in savannah country brings them into close contact with savannah-type tsetse flies, carrier of the acute rhodesian sleeping sickness or, in the forest, to yellow fever-carrying mosquitoes.

People come to recognize danger areas and may prevent exposure or take positive action to eliminate the danger such as draining swamps to prevent mosquito breeding or, in a more modern version, apply insecticides. Vaccination and the production of specific therapeutic chemicals are all cultural efforts to protect human populations.

The belief that illness is a punishment for wrongdoing is widespread in human society. The attribution of illness to misconduct may have been an early form of social order in development of human society. Among the Ganda of East Africa is a belief that a disease causing swelling of the cheeks, limbs and genitals (elephantiasis?) results from the violation of certain taboos.

Among the Irigwe of Nigeria, men who preside over shrine houses have important authority and ritual obligations upon which Irigwe welfare depends. Obligations also relate to diseases for it is believed that if the shrinekeepers do not fulfill their obligations they will provoke the displeasure of ancestors and spirits and become subject to illness and untimely death.

An example of a combination of culture, beliefs and sex

discrimination is found in rituals where men only participate: medical surveys in some west African countries show that the high sleeping sickness incidence among males is probably due to women's exclusion from sacred groves which, in many areas, are major foci of tsetse fly infestation and therefore potentially of high sleeping sickness risk.

Cultural factors have a great impact on health and human development. Attitudes determine the value placed on health by a community, and may therefore decide the request for health services and the use made of them.

Cultural beliefs should be respected, studied and, if possible, understood by all workers in the community. Some beliefs are harmless to health and development and can actually help in programming; others are harmful and long-term educational programs may be needed to effect change. These programs should be planned and implemented with the participation of the people to whom they are directed. Change implies the substitution of one thing for another and every effort should be made to ensure that the advice given is scientifically sound as well as culturally acceptable.

References

Dunn, F. L. (1968) "Epidemiological factors: health and disease in hunter-gatherers", In: "Man the Hunter", R. B. Lee and I. de Vore (eds.), Chicago: Aldine.

Dunn, F. L. (1972) "Intestinal parasitism in Malayan aborigines (Orang Asli)", Bulletin World Health Organization, 46: 99–113.

Gaitskell, A. (1959) Gezira: a story of development in the Sudan. London: Faber & Faber.

Lambrecht, F. L. (1972) "Field studies of Glossina morsitans West. in N'Gamiland, Botswana, in relation to rhodesian sleeping sickness", Bulletin Entomological Research, 62: 183–193.

Lambrecht, F. L. (1981) "Development and diseases in the tropics", International Development Research Centre (Canada), 9: 4–6.

Landy, E. (ed.) (1986) "Culture, Disease and Healing", MacMillan Co., Inc., New York.

Moore, P. D. (1981) "Life seen from a medieval latrine", Nature, 294: 614.

Obeng, L. E. (1969) Man-made Lakes. Accra: Ghana University Press.

Peterson, R. D. and F. L. Lambrecht (1975) "Mosquito breeding related to water storage practices in East-Central State, Nigeria", World Health Organization/VBC/76.647.

Peterson, R. D. and F. L. Lambrecht (1975) "Mosquito breeding in plant axils and tree holes in East-Central State, Nigeria", World Health Organization/VBC/76.64.

Scudder, T. (1966) "Man-made lakes and population resettlement in Africa", In: Man-made Lakes, R. J. Lowe-McConnell (ed.), London: Academic Press for Institute of Biology.

Scudder, T. (1972) "Ecological bottlenecks and the development of the Kariba Lake Basin", In: The Careless Technology. M. T. Favar and J. P. Milton (eds.), New York: Natural History Press.

CHAPTER 11

Elephantiasis: The Curse of Saint Thomas

Frank L. Lambrecht

Written and oral history reveal that elephantiasis, a disease causing swellings of limbs and genitalia, was known from ancient times in many parts of the tropical world. Elephantiasis results from heavy infections with tissue Filaria worms belonging to two different species, *Wuchereria bancrofti* and *Brugia malayi*. The larvae produced by the mature female worms, called microfilariae, live in the bloodstream. Ingested by certain species of mosquitoes, they undergo developmental stages which can re-infect a new human host at the mosquito's subsequent bloodmeals. The breeding places of these mosquitoes are often man-made. Improved sanitation would greatly reduce the number of breeding places and help cut transmission rates. Elephantiasis swellings are caused by the accumulation of adult Filaria worms in certain lymph glands. Because these cutaneous oedemas are permanent disfigurations, traditional medicine has been unsuccessful in dealing with the disease. But so has western medicine. However, the drug diethyl-carbamazine ("Hetrazan") is effective in suppressing the circulation of the worms in the blood stream, thereby reducing the chances of transmission. At present, the drug, together with an effective anti-mosquito campaign, is the most rational means of controlling the disease and reduce its potentials for spread.

History

AMONG THE MANY STORIES BROUGHT BACK BY MARCO Polo, The Venetian world traveller (1254?–1324?), was the ancient legend of Saint Thomas. The apostle, so the tale went, had proven to an Indian King how his belief in the Christian Faith had made it possible for him to perform a miracle by removing single-handed an enormous piece of timber that hindered the shipping along the coast of Malabar. Impressed by such a performance and perceiving the power of a man who could achieve such a miracle, the King granted a large tract of land for the apostle to build a Christian church. But when Saint Thomas' influence and popularity among the inhabitants grew, the King feared the undermining of his own authority. His campaign of harassment and persecution finally forced the apostle to withdraw to the Indian coastal town of Muylepur. Here, one day, he was killed by mistake by the arrow of a low-caste hunter. Soon thereafter, the myth began circulating that the mysterious disease among the inhabitants of the Malabar coast which transformed their legs into huge pillars of flesh was, in fact, the curse for Saint Thomas' martyrdom. Later, when elephantiasis cases were frequently seen and reported by the crew of ships calling at the Malabar port of Cochin, the affliction became known as the "Cochin leg" (Laurence, 1970).

Proof of the great antiquity of elephantiasis is found in Buddhist literature dating between 600 and 250 B.C. referring to the deformity of limbs of the inhabitants along the Ganges River. The disease is mentioned in the two oldest Indian medical studies going back to the 4th century A.D., and in Persian medical literature from the 10th century A.D. Elephantiasis-like swellings of the lower limbs are seen in the statue of the Egyptian Pharaoh Mentuholep (±2000 B.C.). Elephantiasis was regarded a typical disease of the Upper Nile Valley by the Roman poet and philosopher, T. Lucretius Carus

(96–55 B.C.). Elephantiasis was generally well known on the shores of the Mediterranean at the beginning of the Christian Era.

Surviving oral history indicates that elephantiasis existed from ancient times in a number of Pacific islands. A passage in the journal of Captain Cook mentions that the inhabitants of New Caledonia "are inflicted with enormous swellings and ulcerations of legs and feet." Other explorers confirmed that the disease was common in many Pacific islands (Laurence, 1968).

The disease, widespread in Africa, was introduced in the West Indies through the importation of West African slaves. In Barbados, for instance, an uninhabited island until 1625, a 1726 survey indicated a great number of elephantiasis cases among both African and European settlers. Throughout the West Indies the disease became known as the "Barbados leg."

Etiology

Elephantiasis, a term now generally used to describe the clinical aspects of the disease, is caused by the accumulation of adult Filaria worms in certain lymph nodes of the human body. This results in pathological changes, inflammatory reactions and progressive obstruction of lymphatic channels by scar tissue. Common sites of the formation of elephantoid tissue are: the genitalia, the mammary glands, the lymph nodes of the extremities, and the retroperitoneal tissues about the kidneys. After an initial inflammatory phase with acute lymphangitis accompanied by fever, the disease may progress toward the obstructive phase with clinical manifestations of lymph varices, swelling of the scrotum, hydrocele and chyluria, ending into true elephantiasis with enormous swellings of legs, arms, scrotum, mammae or vulva. The thickening of the skin and tissues are permanent pathological changes. They are not absorbed even after the infection has run its course when the adult filariae have reached their maximum life span, perhaps as long as 20 years, and the carrier has not become re-infected which, in itself, is unlikely if he or she lives in endemic area.

Elephantiasis is caused by filaria worms. The life cycle of these parasites starts with the continual production by the mature female worms called microfilariae which circulate with the bloodstream. The worms are eaten by mosquitoes. When the infected mosquito bites a person the mature larvae are deposited on the bite wound and, penetrating into the sub-cutaneous tissues, start circulating with the patient's blood-stream until they accumulate in the lymph nodes. Here they mature into male and female adult worms, a process that takes from 8 to 12 months.

This abbreviated account of the filarial life cycle represent by far not the complete epidemiological picture of the disease. First of all, the two species of Filaria worms involved, occupy different geographical regions: *B malayi* with a patchy dis-tribution essentially in the Far East, *W. bancrofti* solidly represented in the rest of the tropical world. The two Filaria are transmitted by different kinds of mosquitoes. Further-more, while *W. bancrofti* is human-dependent, *B. malayi* also occurs in a wide range of animals, including domestic animals. The picture is further complicated by geographical strain differences which manifest themselves in the time of the 24-hour day during which the microfilariae appear in their great-est numbers in the peripheral blood of the human host. A strain is said to be nocturnal when the peak of microfilariae occurs between 10 pm to 4 am; subperiodical when numbers do not show predominance over the 24-hour period; or diur-nal if the peak occurs during the daylight hours. Fascinatingly, the microfilariae peak in a given area coincides with the peak of biting activity of the regional vector(s). In other words, there seems to have been a hereditary selection of strains adapted to the biting behavior of the local mosquito species which insures maximal chances of transmission of the parasite.

The main vector of bancroftian filariasis, is a mosquito widely distributed in the warm regions of the world. The larvae are found in a wide variety of breeding places, small or large, but especially in water highly polluted with organic matter commonly found in unsanitary human environments. The close association with human habitats, accounts for the major role played by this mosquito in the epidemiology of the disease. Although other mosquitoes, are able to transmit filaria worms, their epidemiological implications vary regionally.

Malayian filariasis is transmitted mainly by mosquitoes belonging to the genera *Mansonia*. The ecology of these mosquitoes is somewhat peculiar in that the larvae depend upon the presence of certain green aquatic plants such as water lettuce and water hyacinth, onto which they attach themselves to secure their supply of oxygen through special mouthparts modified to pierce the plant's stem. Endemic *B. malayia* areas will, therefore, coincide with water courses or marshlands where these plants occur, an association quite different from that of the bancroftian filariasis environment. Another difference, as mentioned above, is that *B. malayia* is found in a number of animals. The role played by animal carriers in the epidemiology of malayian filariasis is uncertain.

As in the case of other mosquito-borne diseases, the potentials of filaria worm transmission are greatly enhanced by man himself through the creation of conditions favoring the proliferation of the mosquito vector. In Sri Lanka, for example, where filariasis increased to dramatic proportions during and after World War II, epidemiological research revealed that some entirely manmade changes, such as the replacement of the traditional pit-latrines in villages along the southwest coast by "modern" septic tank system, may have been responsible for the increase of breeding-places of the mosquito vector, *C. p. fatigans*. It was found that the air-pipe that ventilates the septic tank, was used by the female mosquito to gain entrance for depositing her eggs onto the waste-water below. Moreover, after a while, numerous septic tank covers were cracked or fractured and left unrepaired, giving free access to the female mosquitoes. The country's rapid population increase intensified parasite-man contact in the built-up areas, including the capital Colombo where streets lined with open-drain ditches, often blocked by litter or deterioration, accumulate rain- and wastewater and form permanent puddles ideal to *C. p. fatigans* breeding. Unexpected, amazingly prolific *C. p. fatigans* breeding sites were discovered in earthenware pots filled with water to preserve areca-nuts (betel). Mosquito breeding on an almost industrial scale was observed in huskpits, open-air ponds where the outer shells of coconuts are left to rot in order to separate the fibers later used in the manufacturing of mattresses, mats and ropes. This type of industry is found all along the southwest coast, contributing to the already heavy mosquito infestation in that area. Besides these specific mosquito problems, Sri Lanka is also plagued by those prevalent in other unhygienic tropical environments, with heavy breeding in widespread uncollected refuse of broken bottles, discarded tires, empty cans, and other solid waste paraphernalia (Abdulcader, 1962, '67; Lambrecht, 1971 a & b, 72 & 75).

Due to the great variety of types of breeding places of *C. p. fatigans* and other *W. Bancrofti* and *B. malayia* vectors, the ecology and epidemiology of elephantiasis ranges from strictly urban to completely sylvatic environments, each with its own particular transmission potentials. The Seychelles Islands, where filariasis is of relative recent introduction, is a case in point. When, in 1742, the French landed first in the islands they found the land uninhabited. Commonly associated with man, it is assumed that *C. p. fatigans* was not present in the islands at that time. After the French landing and their later occupation, contact between Seychelles and the outside world was mainly with islands Mauritius, Reunion and Madagascar whence most of the first settlers and later immigrants came, consisting of French colonialists and African laborers. Filariasis may have been introduced by these first inhabitants. At the start lacking the stimulus for rapid expansion, the disease later escalated as a result of the growing population and urbanization which, in turn, provided more breeding opportunities for peridomestic mosquitoes. One may even argue that the introduction and increase of canned food imports, the yield from available arable land being insufficient to feed the population—and the negligent disposal of the empty containers—have contributed to the rapid spread and multiplication of *C. p. fatigans*. Even as late as 1935 was *C. p. fatigans* reported to be rare except in the neighborhood of Port Victoria, the capital city of Mahe, the main island. A 1968–69 survey, however, revealed that the species was one of the most common mosquitoes in the islands (Lambrecht 1971c).

Filiariasis was mentioned for the first time in the 1926 Annual Medical Report with the listing of four cases. Clinical cases of elephantiasis and lymphadenitis were mentioned for the first time in the 1934 Report. In 1969, the filariasis infection rate for Mahe stood at 3.6 percent in a total population of 40,000. However, the rates varied from 3 percent in Port Victoria on the east coast to 25 percent in Port Glaud, a small agricultural village on the west coast (Lambrecht, 1971c). The uneven distribution may be an indication that the disease is still in phase of expansion, active foci, such as Port Glaud, providing maximum conditions for intense transmission. It was also noted that a number of male inhabitants of Port Glaud were contract workers engaged for one or more years to work in the coconut plantations of the Chagos islands where high infection rates of about 20 percent had been found during a 1969 survey. The contact between these two foci could be mutually accumulative (Lambrecht, 1973). Whereas 53 percent of mosquito breeding in Port Victoria area occurred in peridomestic sites, most mosquitoes collected at Port Glaud came from irrigation canals, seepage pools and other sylvatic places (Lambrecht, 1971c).

An unusual mosquito breeding site is that of the new species, *Aedes lambrechti* (Van Someren, 1971) whose larvae were collected uniquely in crab holes. Adult female *A. lambrechti* were found to harbor non-human microfilariae. Another unexpected, prolific source of mosquito breeding were the flower vases on the headstones of the large Port

Victoria cemetery. Because of the high rainfall (about 100 inches annually) during most of the year (average of 18 days of rain per month) these vases and similar rain-catching ornaments, with accumulated debris from flowers and leaves—always contained larvae, including those of *C. p. fatigans*, (Lambrecht, 1971c).

The high rainfall, keeping mosquito breeding sites active year-around, the constant high humidity which promotes long life-span of *C. p. fatigans*, resulting in a high survival rate of the parasite within the insect, and the large amount of peridomestic and other man-made mosquito breeding sites, are major contributing factors in Seychelles filariasis problem (Lambrecht, 1971c).

Disease and Culture

Jacques May (1970) defines disease as a maladjustment of living cells to their environment. Diseases arise with the convergence at a certain time of the pathogenic organism and the human host, and the immunity reaction of the individual. These challenges and responses are not the same in every circumstance. They vary with the geographical and cultural location. The response is conditioned by the genetic make-up of the host. Challenges and response are closely linked to a set of human behavior and customs encompassed in the word "culture."

Culture influences disease occurrence in three main ways: (1) by linking or separating disease agents and host; (2) by changing the environment; (3) by changing the host's response.

Through the choice of location, the inhabitants of a village are facing the challenge of the conditions characterizing that environment, including disease-causing organisms and their vectors. They build their houses according to the style, plan and materials learned from their ancestors. Their occupation, diet and behavior is based upon that of previous generations which has made possible the survival of the group in spite of disease challenges. But cultural traits that were originally acquired for the purpose of survival may outlast its usefulness. Under changing circumstances it may even become detrimental.

A group may decide to migrate but the cultural trait which had been successful in a certain area may prove inappropriate to face the challenges of the new location. Examples of relocations show the traumatic outcome, psychologic as well as physiologic, of such moves. Equally forceful is the impact of the move of rural populations to urban centers where they face a new set of lifestyle and disease patterns.

Cultural changes, often prompted by social and technical evolution, have greatly modified the natural environment in many regions of the world. The impact upon health from the building of a dam and irrigation system, changes in agricultural techniques and crops, modification in water supply and waste disposal have been discussed in another chapter of this volume.

Inspired by his culture, man may disrupt his relationship with a disease agent by taking specific anti-parasite drugs with—hopefully—beneficial effects to himself; vaccination programs protect a large section of the population against certain specific diseases by enhancing or initiating immune response against the disease. The ultimate success of such a technique has been the eradication of small-pox. On the other side, new techniques have introduced extremely harmful compounds, previously non-existent in the environment, such as cancer-causing chemicals and radiation fall-out.

Isolated tribal communities depend upon the resources available where they live and on the knowledge to use them which is passed on by education and training in cultural skills. The traditional healer who accumulates—preserves, so to speak—traditional knowledge within his memory is, therefore, a most important person treated with great respect—and fear—by the members of the community. The traditional healer's training and skills are based on oral tradition inherited from previous generations of "medicine men." His approach to curing a sick person is entirely different from that taken by modern medicine.

Modern medicine considers the sick person as being the object of the illness, a result from infection by micro-organisms, the victim of circumstances, the inheritor of an unfortunate set of genes. The initiation and participation in the treatment is prescribed by the doctor or the surgeon. Non-western medicine emphasizes the sick person as being an actor to be counselled, prompted and enjoined in the healing process. Rituals, ceremonies, drumming, fasting, the use of narcotic or psychedelic substances, and the use of trance are frequently part of the method.

In societies where ill-health is considered a retribution by some evil spirit, the unrelenting swellings of the elephantiasis patient must be particularly heartbreaking to the local witch doctor. The same frustrations confront the professional tradi-tional healer whether his art is based upon Ayurveda, Yunani or Chinese medicine. With the complete failure to find a cure or even alleviate the symptoms of elephantiasis, the tradi-tional medical practitioner had no choice but to declare the disease incurable. Traditional healers have achieved success in curing a number of diseases, by chance or through the finding of an authentic remedy; in elephantiasis cases they had to avow their incompetence in the face of a disease so strange and resilient that it scorned the best prepared remedies.

The "un-natural" behavior of the disease makes the patient a somewhat special person and may explain that, in general, there is no social stigma against him. Besides occasional head-aches, and handicapped as to certain types of work, the ele-phantiasis victim is not a sick patient and may lead an otherwise quite normal life. When severe swelling prohibits work and other activities, the patient is taken care of by his relatives or other villagers.

In India, elephantiasis was attributed to wind, bile or phlegm. For treatment, the Indian physician used blood-letting, also recommended by certain Greek and Roman phy-sicians, or various kinds of plasters, ointments and heat. The patient was advised to fast or to drink caster oil mixed with cow-urine for a month, or take laxatives. If swellings persisted more than a year, the disease was regarded as incurable. Interestingly, some of the Indian scripts mention that the disease occurs especially in swampy places with stagnant water.

The association of elephantiasis with dampness is also be-lieved in some of the Pacific islands. In the Society Islands, the view is still wide-spread that the disease may be transmit-ted by the urine of an elephantiasis patient. In Fiji, diseases in general are thought to be caused by external influences which may be generated by gods or spirits often as punishment for having violated a taboo—medicine is magico-religious. More specific causes for elephantiasis are said to be: walking early morning in heavy dew, wearing wet clothing, frequent contact with water, transmission from parents or the result from inju-ries. The disease was commonly considered incurable but in order to appease the patient, a concoction was prescribed, made from the bark of various "medicinal" trees. During the treatment, the patient had to refrain from eating crab. An-other treatment was the application of massage with coconut oil mixed with certain leaves. In Tahiti, elephantiasis is treated by washing the body with a water extract of the bark of three different trees mixed with coconut oil scented with sandalwood, the root of a secret herb, and the water of a green coconut (Hoeppli, 1959).

Control of Elephantiasis

If elephantiasis is impervious to treatment by traditional medicine, so it is to that by western medicine; once the elephantiasis phase has set in, there is no cure to reverse the process. The only way swellings can be removed or reduced is by surgery of the superfluous tissues, if their locations permits such surgical intervention.

The mosquito vector being a crucial link in the transmission of filariasis, the elimination of its breeding places would greatly reduce transmission rates. A good part of mosquito control can be achieved by simple means of sanitation but one which requires sustained cooperation between inhabitants, and between them and medical authorities. Individual protection against nocturnal filariasis can be gained by sleeping under a mosquito net—also effective against malaria.

The control of transmission by mass chemotherapy has failed in many areas because the only available drug, diethylcarbamazine ("Hetrazan"), is to be administered under medical supervision. It is an anthelminthic that requires repeated doses, sometimes producing serious side reactions in heavily infected patients. In endemic *B. malayia* zones there is the problem of an animal reservoir with risks of re-infections even after the successful treatment of the human carriers. Of course, the early detection of infections through the finding of microfilariae in the bloodstream of carriers during a general survey of the population—and the treatment of the positive cases with diethylcarbamazine—may forestall the build-up of adult filaria worms thereby preventing the lymphatic involvement that gives rise to elephantiasis swellings. Such a campaign—early detection and treatment—combined with an active anti-mosquito program will be the most effective way to reduce elephantiasis in a region. Such an effort can only succeed when supported by an effective collaboration between medical authorities and community leaders and the inhabitants, stimulated by a sustained public health education program. There are such areas where filariasis has disappeared as a result of the improvement of housing standards and a decrease of exposure to mosquito bites through personal prevention or environmental changes that eliminated sources of mosquito breeding. In other places, the disease was controlled as an indirect benefit of malaria control campaigns which indiscriminately affected both the malaria and filariasis vectors. In some Pacific islands where mass chemotherapy has been successfully supervised, transmission of filariasis was completely interrupted.

References

Abdulcader, M. H. M. (1962) "Introduction of filariasis in Ceylon," Journal of Tropical Medicine & Hygiene, 65 (1–2):298–301.

Abdulcader, H. M. H. (1967) "The significance of the *Culex pipiens fatigans*, Wideman, problem in Ceylon," Bulletin World Health Organization, 37:245–249.

Hoeppli, R. (1959) "Parasites and Parasitic Infections in Early Medicine and Science," University of Malaysia Press, Singapore, 526 pages, 23 plates.

Lambrecht, F. L. (1971) "Entomological assessment of the efficiency of mosquito control in the endemic filariasis belt of Ceylon," World Health Organization, Fil/71.93 and W.H.O./V.B.C./71.312.

Lambrecht, F. L. (1971) "Elephantiasis: the adaptation of *Wuchereria bancrofti* to made-made environment," Conference Environmental Science & International Development, Philadelphia, Pennsylvania.

Lambrecht, F. L. (1971) "Preliminary Report on the Distribution and Epidemiology of Filariasis in the Seychelles Islands, Indian Ocean," Southeast Asian Journal Tropical Medicine & Public Health, 2:222–232.

Lambrecht, F. L. & F. B. Fernando (1972) "Mosquito breeding in huskpits compared to other breeding pools of southwest Ceylon," World Health Organization/V.B.C.;72.395.

Lambrecht, F. L. (1973) "Filariasis in the Seychelles Islands and in the British Indian Queen Territories," World Health Organization/FIL/WP/73.3

Lambrecht, F. L. (1975) "Entomological aspects concerning the transmission of *Wuchereria bancrofti*, Cobbold, in Sri Lanka," Bulletin World Health Organization, 51:133–143.

Laurence, B. R. (1968) "Elephantiasis and Polynesian Origin," Nature, Vol. 219, No. 5154:561–563.

Laurence, B. R. (1970) "The Curse of Saint Thomas," Medical History, XIV (4):352–363.

May, J. M. (1970) "The Ecology of Human Diseases," MD Publications, Inc., New York.

Van Someren, E. C. C. (1971) "The description of a new *Aedes* mosquito of the subgenus *Skusea* from the Seychelles," Journal of Entomology (B), 40 (1):21–25.

CHAPTER 12

Childhood Malnutrition in Developing Countries: Integrating Research and Health Care

Stephen G. Sellers

Nutrition programs and malnutrition research in recent decades suggest that programs of the near future will comprehend multiple nutrition interventions and integrate several scientific disciplines.

PROTEIN-ENERGY MALNUTRITION IN INFANCY AND early childhood is a major health problem in most developing countries. It is frequently the principal cause of death, the reason for low life expectancy at birth, and a determinant of retarded growth and development during childhood. The images we usually associate with malnutrition—children with emaciated limbs, swollen bellies, and hollow eyes—are drawn by the news media from occurrences of famine or chronic undernutrition. Efforts directed at combatting protein-energy malnutrition proceed on two fronts: public health programs and scientific investigation. To those of us who work in the field, it sometimes seems as if the two operate at cross-purposes.

In this paper I will suggest that scientific research, particularly behavioral science research, and public policy on issues of malnutrition in developing countries might be better integrated. There are dilemmas in both camps: public health officials cannot wait until all the scientific results are in before acting, nor should they act without informing themselves of the available knowledge (Ordoñez-Pas, 1977); scientists are reluctant to step into volatile political matters yet at other times feel called upon to publicize or even dramatize their results in order to influence policy. Three issues in recent years have presented those sorts of dilemmas and I will review them below. They are: (1) the question of permanent mental impairment caused by early protein-energy malnutrition, (2) the issue of commercial infant formulas and the displacement of breastfeedings, and (3) the effectiveness of direct government interventions to prevent malnutrition through diet supplements. Real differences of opinion have emerged on all these issues, at times argued in the public arena and news services. I will outline here the major points of discussion, note the most recent research findings, and comment on the role of social scientists working on nutrition issues in the near future.

Characteristics of Protein-Energy Malnutrition

Protein-energy malnutrition is due most simply to an insufficient absorption of protein and the other energy sources (fats and carbohydrates) needed to maintain normal metabolic functions. No single amount of nutrients can be prescribed as sufficient because body needs vary with such things as the individual's sex, rate of growth, and level of activity. As an approximate example, 3 year old boys should consume 16 grams of protein and 1,360 Kilocalories of energy for a minimally adequate diet according to guidelines of the World Health Organization and Food and Agriculture Organization of the United Nations, while pregnant women are recommended 34 g protein and 3,090 Kcal (FAO/WHO, 1973). Illness, especially gastrointestinal infection, can be involved with malnutrition in several ways; it may reduce appetite and food intake, diminish nutrient absorption, and increase metabolic demands. Because of the several paths of causality, it has been said that gastrointestinal infection acts synergistically with protein-energy malnutrition (Delgado, et al., 1983).

Health statistics implicate malnutrition in a large proportion of childhood deaths in developing countries. Infant deaths in Guatemala (Table 1), for example were recently 92.5 per 1,000 infants which means that almost 1 in 10 die in the first year of life; of them, 28% die from gastrointestinal infection and/or nutritional deficiencies. In Colombia, Peru, and even Mexico the rates are still almost 50 deaths per 1,000 infants. Rates in the 1 to 4 year-old range are lower, but still high when compared to the United States and also when it is considered that 1 to 4 year-olds should be much more responsive to public health interventions than infants. Precise mortality statistics on malnutrition are not easily available; in part because the poorest countries generally have the highest rates of malnutrition and the least resources for compiling vital statistics, and also because the World Health Organization did not use "protein calorie malnutrition" as a classification code until 1977. This last indicates, too, how recently protein-energy malnutrition was conceptualized as a discrete condition.

Individuals suffering acute malnutrition evidence a number of symptoms and clinical distinction has been made between *kwashiorkor*—typified by swollen or puffy skin especially around the ankles and eyes, shiny or flaky skin, and hair dyspigmentation—and *marasmus*—characterized by extreme

NUTRITION-RELATED CHILDHOOD MORTALITY FOR SELECTED COUNTRIES IN THE AMERICAS

Table shows rates of early childhood mortality and proportion due to malnutrition and gastrointestinal infection. Diarrheal diseases include dysentery, amoebiasis, entiritis, and others. Nutrition includes avitaminosis and others. The World Health Organization did not implement a coding for nutritional marasmus and protein-calorie malnutrition until 1977. Sources for this table are the *United Nations Demographic Yearbook/Annuaire Demographique* for 1980 and 1975.

| | POPULATION | | DEATHS (per 1,000) | | CAUSE OF DEATH (percent) | | | |
	Infants 0–1 yr	Children 1–4 yr	0–1 yr	1–4 yr	Nutrition 0–1 yr	1–4 yr	Diarrhea 0–1 yr	1–4 yr
U.S. (1978)	3,281,000	12,368,000	14.0	0.7	0	1	2	1
Guatemala (1977)	215,310	655,067	92.5	28.8	3	3	25	25
Mexico (1976)	2,620,453	10,205,962	46.8	4.3	1	3	25	25
Colombia (1973)	716,643	2,815,649	47.7	7.0	5	8	20	23
Peru (1972)	474,919	1,726,095	49.4	7.0	4	6	23	27

thinness and the reduction of body fat and muscle (Viteri and Arroyave, 1974). Marasmus is considered a gross caloric deficiency, and is frequently a long-term, or chronic condition; kwashiorkor has been considered a more specific, protein deficiency and the onset may be acute. Pathological conditions like these require medical treatment.

Treatment of the sickest cases, however, is not the most effective method to deal with protein-energy malnutrition. Because a sizeable and predictable portion of the population suffers moderate to severe malnutrition in many developing countries, the illness lends itself to epidemiological treatment; that is, to investigation and prevention in the population at large (DeMaeyer, 1976). Prevention, which deals with causes of malnutrition instead of the consequences, is preferable. The technique that has been developed to measure and monitor the nutritional status of a population is anthropometric. By measuring children's weights and heights and then comparing them to standards derived from well-fed children of the same ages and sex, an evaluation of nutritional status can be made (Keller, Donoso, and DeMaeyer, 1976). The comparison is predicated on our knowledge that an early consequence of undernutrition is retarded physical growth. Substandard height for age is termed "stunting" and substandard weight for height is labelled "wasting" (Waterlow and Rutishauser, 1974). These evaluations are necessarily based on samples that include a large number of children, since each individual child's growth is likely to vary somewhat from the norms.

There is abundant information to demonstrate that protein-energy malnutrition in infancy and childhood is associated with developmental disorders. They include suboptimal physical growth, lessened activity, inferior psychological performance, and—in extreme conditions—death. "Association," however, does not prove causality; it most precisely means that incidents frequently co-occur. The distinction is an important one because, while one might argue that "where there's smoke, there's fire," effective public health interventions require a more precise understanding of how disorders come about. The indisputable correlation of protein-energy malnutrition with developmental problems raises a set of more detailed questions: To what degree do the social environmental factors entailed in poverty underlie both malnutrition and behavioral deficits? At what point(s) does illness intervene to cause or complicate the relationship? Are there critical growth periods during which the body is especially vulnerable to protein-energy malnutrition? Does malnutrition have to reach an especially acute stage to affect growth or behavior? Are developmental deficits permanent or recoverable?

We can now begin to answer some of those questions with more certainty than was possible 15 years ago. This information was unavailable to health officials in the 1960s who strove to design nutrition intervention programs.

Malnutrition and Brain Damage

"Nearly all children among the less privileged populations of underdeveloped countries show retarded growth and development at the time they reach school age; and although they are rarely seriously malnourished during school years, they do not make up for the deficit acquired during preschool years. Recent evidence suggests that the retardation in physical development in infancy is paralleled by impaired mental development, which is probably permanent." (Scrimshaw, 1968)

"Protein deprivation between the ages of six months and a year and one half causes permanent and irreversible brain damage to some young infants." (*Hunger U.S.A.*, quoted in R. Frisch, 1970:189)

In the 1950s and 60s a set of studies on animals and humans by scientists from several disciplines suggested that undernutrition in early childhood caused permanent brain damage. The social significance of such effects would be considerable and, due to government concern and news media reporting, the assumed relationship became widely accepted as proven fact. Research results reported in the 1970s have received less attention, but provide us with a more precise understanding of the process. They indicate that protein-energy malnutrition, even chronic undernutrition, does impair psychological performance, but also that, at least in some circumstances, deficits can be recuperated.

The early studies were of two kinds: (1) animal experiments and (2) retrospective human surveys. Among the first, Dobbing and his colleagues at the University of London found that brain development, myelination, in young rats was significantly impaired when they were experimentally undernourished soon after birth. "It seems likely that the physical growth of the brain can be seriously restricted by comparatively mild undernutrition at the period of its fastest growth, and that such restrictions have permanent sequelae" (1968:200). Extending the animal research to learning, Barnes at Cornell University found that pigs fed grossly deficient protein diets took a significantly longer time to alter learned behavior (Barnes, 1968). Extrapolating from the experimental research with animals, researchers hypothesized that nutritional deficiencies might lead to mental impairment in humans and they gave attention to infancy as the critical period of brain growth and protein as the critically scarce nutrient.

Studies in the 1960s of the psychological performance of children from developing countries who had different nutritional histories, while not providing firm proof, did point in the hypothesized direction. A study of 6 to 11 year-old children in a Guatemalan village reported a significant difference in the "intersensory function" of children from the tallest and shortest height quartiles. The psychological tests, which were designed to tap "intersensory function," involved touching a wooden figure concealed in a box and recognizing its match in a set of viewed cards. The indicator of nutritional status was height-for-age (i.e. evidence of nutritional stunting), the researchers suggested that these results supplied "one more argument that neurological changes present in experimental animals fed grossly deficient diets may have their counterpart in human populations subjected to significant degrees of malnutrition" (Cravioto and Licardie, 1968:266; see also Cravioto, 1966). The shortcoming of such studies was their inability to disassociate nutritional effects on psychological performance from social environmental causes. An impoverished environment leads to nutritional deficiencies and stunting; it may also constrain cognitive development directly and not necessarily by way of malnutrition.

A subsequent set of studies attempted to measure the influence of chronic undernutrition on development in an experimental framework that would control for the confounding effects of social environment. A Guatemalan study provided diet supplements to families from four villages in a region with a high incidence of protein-energy malnutrition. Another study, in poor urban *barrios* of Bogota, Colombia provided food supplements to families at risk of malnutrition (Herrera, et al., 1980). Both programs were multidisciplinary and in both social scientists figured prominently: psychologists to measure children's cognitive performance, sociologists and anthropologists to collect information on childrearing practices and conditions of the social environment. Results from those studies indicate a significant, but moderate, difference in psychological performance between children who received the nutritional supplements and nonsupplemented controls (Waber, et al., 1981; Freeman, et al., 1980). Improvement was generally 4–8% on standard tests of cognitive ability. Those effects are statistically independent of social and economic factors which account for another 5–10% of cognitive test scores.

Results from these investigations and others reported in the last five years allow some further, tentative conclusions on details of the hypothesized relationship between malnutrition and permanent brain damage: (a) lack of protein is less frequently a problem than is total caloric intake; (b) the first 6 months of infancy do not seem to be any more critical than older ages for nutritional influence on growth and psychological development (Lasky, et al., 1981); and (c) nutrition-related intelligence deficits seem to be recoverable, not permanent. The last conclusion is indicated by psychological studies of U.S. children whose social backgrounds were not impoverished but who suffered clinical malnutrition brought on by cystic fibrosis (Lloyd-Still, et al., 1974; Ellis and Hill, 1975) and of Dutch soldiers who had been born just before or during the *hongerwinter* famine of 1944–1945 (Stein, et al., 1972).

Summing up the most recent findings, then, it can be said that the detrimental effects of protein-energy malnutrition on mental development have been confirmed, though impairment is neither so massive nor long-term as was once feared. Overall, the results affirm the remarkable resilience and adaptability of the human body to environmental insult (Stini,

1979). The implications for public health policy are that nutritional interventions are necessary and that, while early intervention is desirable and most effective, it is never too late since impairment may not be irreversible. Dramatizing the possibilities of permanent brain damage in order to instigate a response from policymakers is a device that can backfire: they might be moved to act quickly, but on the other hand they might decide that action is useless on the grounds that remedial intervention would be ineffective.

Infant Formulas

In 1981 the member nations of the World Health Organization voted 118 to 1 to adopt a nonbinding policy restricting the promotion of infant formulas. The United States cast the single dissenting vote explaining that it was unwilling to endorse further governmental imposition on commercial trade and advertising. Afterward, two officials of the U.S. Agency for International Development who had major responsibility for the agency's work on childhood malnutrition in developing countries resigned their posts in protest of the administration's chosen position. To much of the world, and among them many U.S. citizens, it appeared as though the U.S. government was ready to promote international business profit even at the cost of sacrificing infants from developing countries.

The issue of whether public health needs are better satisfied through free commerce or through government edict is one of several that underlies what has been an acrimonious debate between apologists for the multinational companies that manufacture infant formulas and their critics. One reviewer of the controversy has said, "It is a battle in which politics and money, not science, have come to dominate" (Solomon, 1981). The claims and accusations hurled by both sides have hardly advanced the concerted efforts needed to address a real problem: infant weaning syndrome.

In the early 1960s, John Gordon and his colleagues at M.I.T. called attention to a phenomenon they termed "weanling diarrhea." It was characterized by repeated bouts of gastrointestinal infection, usually between the 6th and 18th months of age, after the child had been taken off the breast. When complicated by nutritional deficiencies and other infectious disease, the syndrome often began a downward spiral leading to death. Weanling diarrhea has been implicated in the high infant death rate of most developing nations.

Weaning is a time of particular susceptibility for the child for several reasons. One is that the child's body must shift from a familiar, digestible and nutritious food—mother's milk—to other foods which are unfamiliar, less digestible, and may lack some nutrients. What is more, the introduced foods may contain infectious agents and thereby expose the child to disease. Breastmilk, on the other hand, conveys certain immune agents to the child as Leonardo Mata demonstrated in a longitudinal, etiological study of childhood illness in an Indian village of Quatemala (1978). Infectious disease and intestinal parasites were endemic to the region and Mata carefully analyzed their occurrence in a group of 45 Indian children from their mothers' pregnancies.

Because of the benefits of breastmilk and the risks entailed at weaning, scientists (among them, notably, Margaret Mead (1979)) have documented with concern the worldwide decline in breastfeeding over the last three decades associated with modernization and urbanization (Popkin, 1982). Many viewed with even greater alarm the commercial promotion of infant formulas and bottle feeding in developing countries since they threatened to displace or curtail breastfeeding. One of the foremost researchers to publicize this concern was Derrick Jelliffe who, in 1975, wrote that it was "as yet very little appreciated that the activities of the infant food industry in developing countries in relation to culturally, economically and socially harmful advertising and promotion of inappropriate infant foods needs control, both as regards direct advertising with posters and on the radio and television, and also the more insidious oblique advertising and opinion molding through free samples, networks of milk from nurses and the sponsoring of meetings, etc. by commercial concerns" (Jelliffe, 1975). Reported incidents of mothers unable to breastfeed because their infant had been "hooked" on formula at the hospital, of overdiluted formula causing undernutrition, and of unsanitary and contaminated water used for mixing the formula served to dramatize the injurious effects of commercial infant foods.

One eventual consequence of the concern for these problems was the World Health Organization policy code to restrict infant-formula sales practices. Another was the popular movement in the late 1970s to boycott products made by Nestlé, the Swiss-based food company that commands about one-half the international market for infant formulas. Church and civic groups organized to attempt to coerce Nestlé to publicly acknowledge its past misdeeds and to alter its sales policies.

Extreme statements made by critics of the infant food companies, necessary, perhaps, to rally public support for the issue, tended to exalt breastfeeding and condemn infant formulas. Lost in the exchange of slogans was the simple truth that children must be weaned from the breast at some age and therefore weaning food of some kind is a necessity (Brown, 1978). In fact, since breastfeeding drains the mother's energy reserves, both the infant's and mother's health may be jeopardized among populations at risk of malnutrition by exclusive breastfeeding after the first few months of life. The optimal weaning age has yet to be determined—six months is a frequently cited current guideline—but proper timing must depend upon the mother's nutritional status among other factors.

Research on a number of questions pertaining to this issue call for prompt attention. Must infant formulas supplant breastmilk or can they be complementary? Under what conditions (if any) are commercial infant formulas preferable to local, traditional weaning foods? There is no question that in most circumstances breastfeeding is advantageous to a point, but the fact remains that the necessary transition from breast to grownup diet is an especially sensitive period in child development. The alarm raised about commercial infant formula promotion was certainly warranted, but the response should not obfuscate or deter objective research on breast-feeding and weaning foods. Nor should our renewed recognition of the importance of mother's milk lead us to neglect the real need of many mothers and infants for breast milk substitutes. Politicization of the issues created for time a climate in which it was difficult to carry out scientific research.

The Technological Fix

Proposed technological inventions to reduce worldwide malnutrition, or the so-called "protein gap," flourished in the 1960s. Exotic solutions such as harvesting whales and manatee, ocean farming of algae, synthesizing meat substitutes from soybean, plant breeding high-yielding grains, amino acid fortification of cereals, and producing single-cell protein on a petroleum base are among the imaginative suggestions.

It is understandable that there are numerous proposals to "cure" protein-energy malnutrition given the remarkable success of medical research in this century to invent cures and preventive techniques for centuries-old maladies. The dramatic reduction of cholera through sanitary water treatment, of typhoid and yellow fever by innoculation, and of malaria through DDT mosquito eradication have generated an appealing model for epidemiological health care. Analogous proposals to discover a technological solution for protein-energy malnutrition include grain fortification, inexpensive dietary supplements, nutrition education, birth control, and the breeding of high-yield crops. Experience over the last two decades has shown that each of these has some merit, yet no single technique offers the promise of eradicating protein-energy malnutrition. Food fortification, though a proven success for preventing goiter with iodine and a promising technique for dealing with vitamin A deficiency, does not appear to be a practical measure for combatting protein deficiencies (Austin, 1979).

The case of diet supplements, which attempt directly to combat malnutrition, is especially instructive. Feeding programs have been conducted in a number of developing countries; among them are India, Pakistan, New Guinea, Haiti, Dominican Republic, Colombia, Costa Rica, and Guatemala. The nature of these programs varies in many ways: (a) the size and composition of the client population; whether it is rural or urban, local or regional, or focuses on a targeted subset of the population; (b) the form of food supplement which can be specially developed formulas, donated food surpluses, or augmentation of customary foods; (c) the composition of supplements varying in protein, energy, and other nutrients; (d) the method of distribution, sometimes at nutrition rehabilitation centers, delivered to the home, or distributed from a central location; and (e) other programmatic interventions accompanying food supplementation as, for example, home instruction, medical care, and community organization.

It is not easy to reach general conclusions from supplementation programs because comparisons are complicated by the many differences in detail. Furthermore, the absence of appropriate control subjects or comparative data in many programs, qualifies the validity of the results. Several recent comparative reviews of program results (Martorell, et al., 1976; Anderson et al., 1981; Beaton and Ghassemi, 1982; Gwatkin, Wilcox, and Wray, 1980) however permit some general conclusions.

Most studies report a beneficial impact of supplementation on children's physical growth, the usual indicator of nutritional status, and several report a reduction in infant mortality. Response to supplementation tended to be greatest among the youngest children and those most deficient in weight for height (Martorell and Klein, 1980; Gopalan, et al., 1973). Combined protein and calorie supplements are generally most effective, though one review (Martorell, et al., 1976) suggests that the relative benefit depends on which nutrients are most limiting in the usual home diet.

Of equal significance to these findings is the fact that no supplementation programs reported an absolute elimination of mild-moderate malnutrition, although several had a significant impact on preventing the incidence of severe malnutrition. It should also be noted that in some programs the benefits of supplementation were enhanced by medical treatment of infection (Kielmann, Taylor, and Parker, 1978), and by early childhood education (McKay, et al., 1978). These results suggest that, depending on local conditions, a multi-faceted approach is probably most effective in dealing with malnutrition and its sequelae. In Bogota, for example, a home education program in which the mother was taught educational activities to play with the child, did not by itself improve children's diet or growth, but it did enhance the benefits of supplementation for both diet intake and physical growth (Mora, et al., 1981; Overholt, et al., 1982).

Program effectiveness can be measured with several outcome measures; among them are mortality, physical growth, amount of supplement consumed, net increment in nutrient adequacy, and behavior. All these measures can be informative, but may lead to different conclusions about program effectiveness. Perhaps the major criterion considered by policymakers in evaluating effectiveness is cost/benefit. This reasoning is neither callous nor mercenary, but rather a recognition of the scarcity of public health funds in developing countries; budget constraints make it imperative that resources be utilized in ways that will yield the most good. One program review concludes that "food distribution programs directed toward young children, as now being operated, are rather expensive for measured benefit" (Beaton and Ghassemi, 1982). The authors point out, however, that some program benefits may go unrecognized, for example sharing of food with non-participants and income substitution by poor families.

Food supplement costs are not irrelevant. The hoped-for benefit of Incaparina, a high protein/low-cost grain meal developed at the Institute of Nutrition of Central America and Panama in the early 1960s and marketed by the Quaker Oats Company, was largely unrealized because it was still too expensive for the poorest and neediest Guatemalan families. Much of the cost/benefit effectiveness of food supplementation programs, then, may be contingent on subsidization by a government or relief agency. Subsidization, in turn, is sometimes a short-term exigency but may be an unreliable long-term solution to protein-energy deficits.

Food supplements are illustrative of a number of the public health issues that arise in dealing with malnutrition. They have some demonstrable benefits, but we should not be tempted to view diet supplementation as *the* solution to malnutrition.

Conclusions

The most significant realization of the 1970s was that appropriate technologies were necessary, but not sufficient mechanisms to accomplish major reductions in protein-energy malnutrition. One scientist who has devoted his career to the problem has written candidly in this regard

> "As a biologist and student of public health I cannot avoid recognizing the health problems of the village and other similar localities and asking if feasible solutions can be evolved and implemented. However, the danger exists in the tendency of health professionals to assess the problem from the single biological viewpoint, often the first step in a series of errors. What the biologist overlooks is that the individual he examines is a member of a society in which 50 percent of the people are illiterate, sanitary provisions are inadequate, housing is deficient, and nutrition is poor . . . To recommend interventions capable of improving health and growth of village children calls for responsibility and careful analysis." (Mata, 1978:324)

Many of the most sensational proposals and the most alarming hypotheses have turned out to be less extreme than was originally suspected. This in itself constitutes progress both for science and public health, and it has been achieved through research. Whether the dramatization of initial claims has helped the effort by attracting public attention and research funds or has hindered it by diverting researchers and policymakers from objective investigation is a debatable issue. I am persuaded that the latter, unfortunately, has been the predominant effect.

Foreign and development assistance aimed at nutrition health care has evolved through different stages in recent decades. In the 1950s much of the effort was diagnostic involving clinical observations at health care centers and epidemiological surveys in the field. These efforts achieved an initial conceptualization of the manifestations and magnitude of malnutrition. Treatment in those years was largely hospital-based and relied especially on the transfer of technologies from developed countries. In the 1960s, the recognition that transferred technologies were frequently unsuited to the circumstances of developing, tropical countries, promoted localized research and invention in areas such as food production, environmental engineering, and family planning. The aspiration in the 1960s was that appropriate technologies could overcome the food and nutrition problems of developing countries. In the 1970s a number of those technologies were adopted by national governments and by international development agencies. In several countries large-scale programs were implemented, often managed by native professionals and sponsored by international development loans. At the same time, and sometimes in conjunction with them, field experiments were conducted to evaluate the effectiveness of interventions.

Social scientists have figured in nutrition efforts at all stages: sociologists and anthropologists in the field surveys of the 50s, economists in the development projects of the 60s, psychologists and other behavioral scientists in the applied research projects of the 70s. At all stages, however, the participation tended to be project-specific just as the projects were intervention-specific; that is, an anthropologist's assigned task might be to discover prevailing weaning customs within the context of a program directed toward lactating mothers. Such a topic was certainly pertinent to childhood malnutrition, but unless integrated into a broader programmatic approach it had little likelihood of leading to significant improvement.

As the 1980s get underway we now find ourselves reevaluating the accomplishments and failures of the past decades. One common assessment is that institutional changes will be required in many countries in order to realize a greater social benefit from technological innovations. Despite increased agricultural production high rates of protein-calorie malnutrition persisted in most developing countries through the 1970s; the neediest did not reap their requisite share from improved harvests. A meeting of Latin American health officials in 1981 concluded that "although food production was essential, that in itself could not solve basic hunger and malnutrition. Food strategies should also take into account those economic and social policies affecting food consumption and distribution, and income distribution" (United Nations, 1981). It also seems likely that, for the proximate future at least, nutrition health programs cannot expect to eliminate malnutrition with a preestablished intervention. Instead comprehensive programs will be organized so as to evolve in assessing and addressing health conditions as they change. The one-shot solution will not work. In the *barrios* of many Latin American cities, potable water and sanitary waste disposal might receive the initial priority, as the most cost-effective method to reduce malnutrition and, once implemented, might be followed by ensuring dietary intake or modifying weaning practices. I am not attempting to prescribe a set plan, however; but rather to illustrate how an agency must contain the capability to design and evaluate multiple strategies. Programs will have to be developed on site and will continuously monitor conditions in order to decide the next most effective line of attack. There is now a much greater appreciation of the fundamental importance to malnutrition of the social-cultural environment and a heightened receptivity to social scientists as integral members of nutrition teams (Berg, 1973). In the current decade we will

178   STEPHEN G. SELLERS

be challenged to demonstrate the utility of social science
techniques for such things as identifying optimal points of
intervention, selecting appropriate preventive strategies, and
evaluating program impacts in comprehensive malnutrition
programs. Our success will be judged by the coming generation of public health professionals.

References

Anderson, Mary Ann, James Austin, Joe Wray, and Marian Zeitlin
    (1981) "Supplementary Feeding." Pp. 25–48 in Harvard Institute
    for International Development (J. Austin, project director), Nu-
    trition Intervention in Developing Countries: An Overview. Cam-
    bridge: Oelgeschlager, Gunn and Hain Publisher.
Austin, James (1979) "Cereal Fortification: An Overview." Pp. 1–14
    in J. Austin (ed.), Global Malnutrition and Cereal Fortification.
    Cambridge: Ballinger Publishing.
Barnes, Richard, A. U. Moore, Ian Reid, and Wilson Pond (1968)
    "Effects of Food Deprivation on Behavioral Patterns." Pp. 203–
    217 in Nevin Scrimshaw and John Gordon (eds.), Malnutrition,
    Learning, and Behavior. Cambridge: MIT Press.
Beaton, G. H., and H. Ghassemi (1982) Supplementary Feeding
    Programmes for Young Children in Developing Countries, Sup-
    plement to American Journal of Clinical Nutrition 35(4).
Berg, Alan (1973) The Nutrition Factor: Its Role in National De-
    velopment. Washington, D.C.: The Brookings Institution.
Brown, Roy (1978) "Weaning Foods in Developing Countries."
    American Journal of Clinical Nutrition 31:2066–2072.
Cravioto, Joaquín (1966) "Malnutrition and Behavioral Develop-
    ment in the Pre-School Child." Pp. 74–84 in National Academy of
    Sciences—National Research Council, Pre-School Child Mal-
    nutrition: Primary Deterrent to Human Progress. Washington,
    D.C.: National Academy of Sciences.
Carvioto, Joaquín, and Elsa R. de Licardie (1968) "Intersensory
    Development of School-Age Children." Pp. 252–268 in Nevin
    Scrimshaw and John Gordon (eds.), Malnutrition, Learning, and
    Behavior. Cambridge: MIT Press.
Delgado, Hernán, Victor Valverde, José Belizán, and Robert Klein
    (1983) "Diarrheal Diseases, Nutritional Status, and Health Care:
    Analyses of their Interrelationship." Ecology of Food and Nutri-
    tion 12:229–234.
DeMaeyer, E. M. (1976) "Protein-Energy Malnutrition." Pp. 23–54

in G. H. Beaton and J. M. Bengoa (eds.), Nutrition in Preventive Medicine: The Major Deficiency Syndromes, Epidemiology, and Approaches to Control. Geneva: World Health Organization.

Dobbing, John (1968) "Effects of Experimental Undernutrition on Development of the Nervous System." Pp. 181–202 in Nevin Scrimshaw and John Gordon (eds.), Malnutrition, Learning, and Behavior. Cambridge: MIT Press.

Ellis, Edward C. and Donald E. Hill (1975) "Growth, Intelligence, and School Performance in Children with Cystic Fibrosis who have had an Episode of Malnutrition during Infancy." Journal of Pediatrics 87(4):565–568.

FAO/WHO (1973) Energy and Protein Requirements. Rome: Food and Agriculture Organization of the United Nations.

Freeman, Howard, Robert Klein, John Townsend, and Aaron Lechtig (1980) "Nutrition and Cognitive Development Among Rural Guatemalan Children." American Journal of Public Health 70(12):1277–1285.

Frisch, Rose (1970) "Present Status of the Supposition that Malnutrition Causes Permanent Mental Retardation." American Journal of Clinical Nutrition 23(2):189–195.

Gopalan, C., M. C. Swaminathan, V. K. Krishna Kumari, D. Hanumantha Rao, and K. Vijayaraghavan (1973) "Effect of Calorie Supplementation on Growth of Undernourished Children." American Journal of Clinical Nutrition 26:563–566.

Gwatkin, Davidson, Janet Wilcox, and Joe Wray (1980) "The Policy Implications of Field Experiments in Primary Health and Nutrition Care." Social Science and Medicine 14C:121–128.

Herrera, M. G., J. O. Mora, N. Christiansen, N. Ortiz, J. Clement, L. Vuori, D. Waber, B. de Paredes, and M. Wagner (1980) "Effects of Nutritional Supplementation and Early Education on Physical and Cognitive Development." Pp. 149–184 in R. R. Turner and F. Reese (eds.), Life-Span Developmental Psychology. New York: Academic Press.

Jelliffe, Derrick (1975) "Nutrition and Economics in the Modern World." Environmental Child Health 267–269.

Kallen, David (1971) "Nutrition and Society." Journal of the American Medical Association 215(1):94–100.

Keller, W., G. Donoso, and E. M. DeMaeyer (1976) "Anthropometry in Nutritional Surveillance: A Review Based on Results of the WHO Collaborative Study on Nutritional Anthropometry." Nutrition Abstracts and Reviews 46(8):591–609.

Kielmann, Arnfried, Carl Taylor, and Robert Parker (1978) "The Narangwal Nutrition Study: A Summary Review." American Journal of Clinical Nutrition 31:2040–2052.

Lasky, Robert, Robert Klein, Charles Yarbrough, Patrician Engle, Aaron Lechtig, and Reynaldo Martorell (1981) "The Relationship between Physical Growth and Infant Behavioral Development in Rural Guatemala." Child Development 52:219–226.

Lloyd-Still, John, Irving Hurwitz, Peter Wolff, and Harry Shwachman (1974) "Intellectual Development after Severe Malnutrition in Infancy." Pediatrics 54:306–311.

McKay, Harrison, Leonardo Sinisterra, Arlene McKay, Hernando Gomez, and Pascuala Lloreda (1978) Improving Cognitive Ability in Chronically Deprived Children. SCIENCE 200; 270–278.

Martorell, Reynaldo and Robert Klein (1980) "Food Supplementation and Growth Rates in Preschool Children." Nutrition Reports International 21(3):447–454.

Martorell, Reynaldo, Aaron Lechtig, Charles Yarbrough, Hernán Delgado, and Robert Klein (1976) "Protein-Calorie Supplementation and Postnatal Physical Growth: A Review of Findings from Developing Countries." Archivos Latinoamericanos de Nutrición 26(2):115–128.

Mata, Leonardo (1978) The Children of Santa María Cauqué: A Prospective Field Study of Health and Growth. Cambridge: The MIT Press.

Mead, Margaret (1979) "Family Contexts of Breastfeeding." Pp. 3–24 in Dana Raphael (ed.), Breastfeeding and Food Policy in a Hungry World. New York: Academic Press.

Mora, José O., Stephen Sellers, Jorge Suescún, and M. Guillermo Herrera (1981) "The Impact of Supplementary Feeding and Home Education on Physical Growth of Disadvantaged Children." Nutrition Research 1:213–225.

Ordoñez-Paz, Antonio (1977) "Pragmatic Aspects of Program Evaluation Regarding Child Care and its Relation to Decisionmaking at the Political-Administrative Level." Pp. 47–55 in J. Bosch and J. Arias (eds.), Evaluation of Child Health Services: The Interface between Research and Medical Practice. Washington, DC: U.S. Department of Health, Education, and Welfare publication #78–1066.

Overholt, Catherine, Stephen Sellers, José O. Mora, Belén de Paredes, and M. Guillermo Herrera (1982) "The Effects of Nutritional Supplementation on the Diets of Low-Income Families at Risk of Malnutrition." American Journal of Clinical Nutrition 36:1153–1161.

Popkin, Barry, Richard Bilsborrow, and John Akin (1982) "Breast-Feeding Patterns in Low-Income Countries." Science 218:1088–1093.

Scrimshaw, Nevin (1968) "Food." Pp. 502–508 in The International Encyclopedia of the Social Sciences, Vol. 5, New York: McMillan Company.

Solomon, Stephen (1981) "The Controversy over Infant Formula." New York Times Magazine, December 6:92–106.

Stein, Zena, Mervyn Susser, Gerhart Saenter, and Francis Marolla (1972) "Nutrition and Mental Performance." Science 17:708–713.

Stini, William (1979) "Adaptive Strategies of Human Populations under Nutritional Stress." Pp. 387–407 in William Stini (ed.), Physiological and Morphological Adaptation and Evaluation. The Hague: Mouton.

United Nations (1981) "Call for Coherent Food Strategy for Latin America, Caribbean Region." U.N. Monthly Chronicle 18(4):24–25.

Demographic Yearbook/Annuaire Demographique 1980. (1982) New York: United Nations.

Viteri, Fernando, and Guillermo Arroyave (1974) "Protein-Calorie Malnutrition." Pp. 604–624 in R. S. Goodhart and M. E. Shils (eds.), Modern Nutrition in Health and Disease. Philadelphia: Lea and Febirger.

Waber, Deborah, Lea Vuori-Christiansen, Nelson Ortiz, John Clement, Niels Christiansen, José O. Mora, Robert Reed, and M. Guillermo Herrera (1981) "Nutritional Supplementation, Maternal Education, and Cognitive Development of Infants at Risk of Malnutrition." American Journal of Clinical Nutrition 34:807–813.

Waterlow, J. C., and Ingrid Rutishauser (1974) "Malnutrition in Man." Pp. 13–25 in Early Malnutrition and Mental Development, Symposia of the Swedish Nutrition Foundation No. 12, Sweden: Almqvist and Wiksell.

CHAPTER 13

Two Decades of a Nutrition Program in Guatemala: A Policy Analysis of the Incaparina Project

Robert P. Wise

Incaparina inspired great optimism at its inception in 1961. The low cost, high protein mixture of vegetable sources was widely expected to help reduce malnutrition of poverty, providing the food equivalent of meat or milk at about a tenth of the cost. Review of its course in Guatemala reveals commercial success with almost continuous growth of sales, but little impact on the poor. The better educated account for most of its consumption and children for relatively little. Industry structure, technology of manufacture, promotional methods, and price all need to be modified to increase its consumption by the poor.

Introduction

IN GUATEMALA, THE CENTRAL IMPORTANCE OF CHRONIC hunger is clear. It contributes heavily to high death rates at young ages. Only about 20 percent of children under age five years normally nourished, and over 30 percent are moderately or severely starved (Wise, 1982; Plan Nacional, no date; Inter-American Development Bank, 1979).

In the aftermath of Guatemala's change of government in 1954 (with violent reversal of a progressive land reform), scientists at the Institute of Nutrition of Central American and Panamá (INCAP) grappled with the enormity of hunger. Then, by mixing vegetable sources, they thought they had a solution to malnutrition of poverty. They had developed a low cost, high protein formula (later called Incaparina, "INCAP flour" in Spanish, from *harina*) offering the nutritional equivalent of meat or milk at as little as a tenth of the cost. Such a promising approach sparked enthusiasm in the international development community. Never explicit, but neither can it have been far from the surface, was anticipation that this product would not seem to threaten anyone's interests. It should not, for example, provoke resistance from the military or the big landowners. Unlike redistribution of land, a very sensitive issue, mixing by-products of cottonseed oil extraction with ordinary corn meal seemed an innocuous but very promising means to cut the cost of food for the poor.

Factors constraining the nutritional impact of Incaparina in Guatemala have been outlined previously (Wise, 1980). These factors are, essentially, monopoly and inefficiency. The fact that only one company makes this product obstructs in more than one way the realization of Incaparina's potential.

Background

The Institute of Nutrition of Central America and Panamá (INCAP), in Guatemala City, developed the concept of Incaparina from laboratory to commercial production by the national beer monopoly, Cervecería Centroamericana, S.A. Marketing of Incaparina began in 1961. To improve administrative efficiency, a wholly-owned subsidiary, Alimentos, S.A., was subsequently created.

INCAP was administratively part of the Pan American Health Organization (PAHO), which in turn is a regional office of the World Health Organization. But little of INCAP's budget was from PAHO. Instead, most was secured autonomously as research grants and contracts. Only formal approval from PAHO's director was normally supplied to important INCAP decisions, such as periodic renewal of the exclusive license with Cervecería, S.A./Alimentos, S.A. to manufacture Incaparina. In 1978, PAHO staff in Washington were reluctant to perpetuate this arrangement. License renewal was delayed, monthly reporting of manufacturing output to INCAP was curtailed, and word was leaked from the beer factory that Incaparina production would cease if its license was not exclusively renewed. A compromise two-year renewal was finally agreed upon, during which period INCAP was to study further the possibility of demonopolization.

The Paradigm of Three Decision Orders

A useful framework for analyzing nutrition interventions is offered by Montgomery:

> "Since decisions are rarely taken in isolation from immediate political and social events, and since they are both too numerous and varied to be analyzed in exhaustive detail, it is more efficient in considering alternatives in nutrition programs to take up only categories of decisions, and to focus on those that constitute the main dimensions of policy. These categories can be grouped into three major dimensions of decision: first, choices among the technologies to be used in improving the national nutrition status; second, decisions about the organizations and agencies that are to convey the improved food or practices; and third, alternative approaches to providing incentives in order to encourage affirmative responses to the program. These three "orders" or classes of decisions are often made independently in spite of their obvious interconnection, but it is the interaction among them that constitutes the major elements and dynamics of a national nutrition system." (1977:314–315).

Incaparina incorporated the technology choices to create a lower cost alternative food by blending vegetable products, and then to manufacture and package it with machine-intensive processes. The principal implementing organizations were INCAP for product development, the brewery, Cervecería Centroamericana, S.A., and the wholly-owned subsidiary, Alimentos, S.A., for production. Distribution from factor to retailer was reportedly opened to competition (INCAP, 1965). A wide range of retailers handled final distribution, such as supermarkets, urban and rural shops of varying sizes, and even open marketplace stands. Incentives for the poor to use Incaparina were its relatively low price, small packages, and promotion by commercials, INCAP, and the government, with the basic message that this flour would be good for health. These elements of the Incaparina program's first two decades are summarized in Table 1.

Inadequacies of the Incaparina program can be understood in terms of each of these three decision levels: the technology is not optimal, implementing organizations are not satisfactory, and the incentives for consumer participation—for the

Table 1
Incaparina in Guatemala: A Nutrition Program
Characterized in Terms of Three Decision Orders

Technology — Blend low-cost vegetable products to yield an inexpensive alternative to milk, cheese, eggs, and meat.

— Machine-intensive manufacture and packaging

Organizations — INCAP developed the product and continues quality control.

— Cervecería Centroamericana, S.A./Alimentos, S.A. manufactures and packages.

— The free market distributes at wholesale and retail levels.

Incentives — The price is low compared to milk.

— "Affordable"-sized packages

— Promotion appeals to health value.

— (Minor subsidy program)

poor to use Incaparina as a substitute for more expensive animal products—are inadequate.

Technology

The basic concept, blending low cost vegetable sources to yield less expensive products with amino acid balances equivalent to animal protein products, remains sound. But under present production arrangements, the ratio of capital to labor in manufacturing resource inputs is high, the opposite of the socially desirable and efficient arrangement in this Third World setting, with labor surplus and associated low price per unit of labor. From the economic viewpoint, the "least cost rule" predicts that the cheapest way to mix resource inputs is in inverse proportion to their prices: use more of what is cheaper and less of what is more costly. More precisely, at the margin the ratio of each input's price to its marginal revenue product will be the same. So why does the manufacturer of Incaparina not use labor-intensive processes instead of capital-intensive ones? The economist would respond that Cervecería, S.A./Alimentos, S.A. might not be operating in the most efficient possible manner, at the minimum point on its average cost curve, simply because there are no competitors to force price down to marginal cost. In contrast, we would expect introduction of competition or such other forces as downward pressure on price from regulating authorities to lead to an increase in the ratio of employees to machines in fabrication processes.

In like manner we can interpret the packaging in current use, relatively expensive, small, and elaborate, as reflecting absence of competitive forces which would maximize efficiency. In Guatemala, products similar to Incaparina in their potential for fungal and insect infestation and damage are ordinary corn and wheat flours. These flours are sold prepackaged in supermarkets, but in much larger units, such as five pound bags, in contrast to one pound bags and 75 gram (2.6 ounce) envelopes of Incaparina. Moreover, the rural majority of Guatemalans purchase flour in bulk from 100 pound sacks in the marketplace, using their own bags or plain paper or plastic sacks of the merchant. It is thus difficult to justify the technologic choices for Incaparina to use capital-intensive manufacture and packaging. But absence of competitive pressure to maximize efficiency makes the situation understandable and implies that demonopolization would contribute to improvement of the Incaparina program in the future.

Organizations

For the first twenty years of its production, all Incaparina fabrication has been centralized at Cervecería, S.A./Alimentos, S.A. Incaparina's wholesale and retail distribution are also in the private sector. However, except for a brief period after 1961, both of the latter functions have been freely competitive.

In principle, some 24,000 commercial corn millers, "most of whom live round the 'barrios,' or towns, rural villages and hamlets" (Urrutia, *et al.*, 1977), could produce the flour mixture. They, along with agricultural cooperatives, are like actors waiting in the wings to become involved, but they have not yet been able to play a role. Their mills, powered by water or electricity, vary in size, normally grind wheat and corn flours, and are often syndicated commercially with systematic quality control as a consequence.

Agricultural cooperatives continue to enjoy official favor, but they do not play an important role in most areas of the country. Still, they represent another potential organizational alternative for Incaparina production.

Technology choices in past and future inter-related with organizational ones. Under monopoly, there is little marketplace pressure to use the most efficient processes. If, in the future, multiple producers could become active, then a spontaneous, concomitant evolution to more efficient, labor-intensive manufacture would be expected, along with sale of the product in bulk and other less expensive packaging. Small millers as well as cooperatives should be prime candidates to produce Incaparina in the future.

Incentives

For consumers who need cheaper and better food, the incentives to use Incaparina can be strengthened. The poor buy little Incaparina, perceiving it as a substitute for ordinary flour, which is cheaper, and probably believing that the product is very potent, so only a little is needed (Solien de González, 1964). In contrast, literate, urban, middle classes find the attractive red package on their supermarket shelves and understand the promotional messages more completely. (Many rural peasants are Mayan Indians, for whom Spanish is not their first language, if they use it at all.)

Reduction of price would increase demand. Price cuts might be achieved through voluntary (unlikely) or regulated reduction of profit level. But the most reliable way to reduce prices would be through freed-up market forces. When more than a few manufacturers exist, the competitive market pressure alone pushes price down to the level of marginal cost, unless other conditions also required for free competition are not satisfied. Conditions required for a freely competitive market include many small buyers; many small sellers; no barriers to entry; no barriers to exit; a homogeneous, divisible product; and a free flow of good information.

If a subsidy were used to reduce the price of Incaparina, as once attempted on a small scale (CARE, 1976), then the consumer would see a lower price and demand larger quantities. But such distortion of supply and demand would either lead to shortages, or else the subsidy would have to be expensive, if it were large enough to accomplish much. Nonetheless, subsidies might appear attractive from a policy viewpoint (Wise, 1980). Since the elasticity of demand for food is high for the very poor, a decrement in price will cause a disproportionate increment in consumption by the target group (Jul, 1978). In contrast, those with normal ranges of income generally have highly inelastic demand curves for food, so the middle and upper classes would only slightly increase their consumption in response to a price cut. This natural targeting of the benefit of a price reduction is a strong argument in favor of somehow reducing the price of Incaparina.

If the price is dropped through substantial subsidy, then future difficulty in reducing that subsidy may be anticipated. Populations notoriously insist on maintaining their food buying power. In one common pattern, a government decreases food subsidies in response to International Monetary Fund pressure to tighten its budget. Food riots often follow, and in some cases they lead to restored subsidy levels. Accordingly, it would seem far preferable to avoid subsidy from the outset. Instead, where remediable departures from conditions needed for free competition can be identified, as in the case of Incaparina, lower food prices should be achieved by freeing up the marketplace.

Another incentive for the poor to use Incaparina should be information. Promotional efforts in the first twenty years of the Incaparina program have not reached those most in need. In part, the reason might be that the manufacturer, as a profit-maximizer, aims at those with more buying power. To date, advertizing has been characterized by use of print media and the Spanish language. Not surprisingly, then, a highly significant association between education of the housewife and frequency of family consumption of Incaparina (Figure 1) emerged in an INCAP nutrition student's survey of Incaparina consumption in rural areas of Guatemala (Cerón, 1978). But most of those in need of the lower cost alternative to animal products are not educated at all. Four-fifths of mothers and half of fathers in another survey had no education at all (Wise, 1978). This sample was almost entirely Indian, representing both urban and rural groups in Totonicapán, Guatemala.

Taking the likelihood of child death in a family as an index of poverty and of need for Incaparina, this survey also showed that at least one child had died more often among families living further from town, where the health centers are lo-

Figure 1

PERCENTAGE OF FAMILIES USING INCAPARINA
BY MATERNAL EDUCATIONAL LEVEL

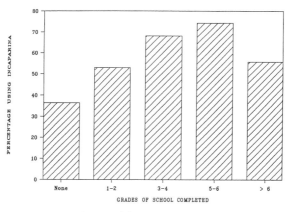

Source of data: Cerón, 1978

cated. This poorer rural health status is no surprise and was statistically very significant. Further, rural dwellers were more likely to be Mayan Indians, and the likelihood of child death was almost three times greater among Indians than in *ladino* families.

Thus, Incaparina promotion has been aimed at those literate in Spanish, but the large majority of housewives and half of men in a Mayan Indian department have no education. The group that needs nutritional assistance tends to live further from town and use Mayan languages, not Spanish.

Promotion of Incaparina in the Quiché language alone would not reach all of the intended beneficiaries. There are three more large Mayan language groups (and about 20 mutually non-intelligible languages in all), and even *ladinos* are often illiterate. But addition of oral promotion, probably by radio, in the various local languages would reach a large fraction of the needy.

The content of publicity about Incaparina also requires improvement. In the past, detailed information has been supplied to the international academic and governmental communities in English and Spanish. But the local populace sees little more than billboards and posters (especially in health centers) with a happy, chubby child and the limited message, *"Incaparina da vigor"* ("Incaparina gives vigor," i.e., health.) The product's name only means "INCAP flour," so in the absence of sustained, oral messages, in intelligible languages, it is not surprising that consumers do not perceive the mixed flour product as a substitute for animal protein products. Rather, they see Incaparina as just another kind of flour, one with a very high price. They do not realize that its price is actually low, enabling them to buy nutrients similar to milk, but at only 10 percent of the cost.

The intended beneficiaries cannot be motivated by incentives they do not understand. Adding better marketplace information in local languages via oral media and with more complete nutritional explanations would not be expensive. However, these changes could be opposed by those whose interests might be threatened. Producers of milk, cheese, eggs, and meat might fear that sales of their products would suffer if the general population learned that a lower cost alternative is available. Whether their sales would in fact fall appreciably is doubtful, since those responding to the message that good quality protein can be found at a lower price would be mainly those who presently consume little of these expensive products. Nonetheless, opposition to efforts to improve the Incaparina program should be anticipated. Reforming efforts will require sufficient support to overcome potential obstructions.

Conclusion

Incaparina consumption estimates based on data reported by Cerón (1978) indicate that only about 6 percent of children below age 12 receive Incaparina daily, in amounts slightly better than one-third of the recommended level. Additional children consume Incaparina at lesser frequencies, but about

87 percent of the youngest group (through age 6) and of seven to eleven year olds receive none.

In the future, much greater impact might be obtained from the still sound concept of vegetable blends as a cheaper source of animal quality protein foods. Decentralization of manufacture and more labor-intensive production and packaging would increase output and reduce prices. More complete flows of information to the target populations would also be expected to contribute to an important increase in consumer demand.

Disclaimer

This chapter reflects work completed before the author assumed his position at the Food and Drug Administration. His views are not necessarily those of the FDA.

References

CARE (1976) Evaluation of the Incaparina Program by CARE. Unpublished.

Cerón de Castañeda, Dalia Margarita (1978) Consumo de Incaparina a Nivel Familiar. Thesis, Instituto de Nutrición de Centro América y Panamá and Universidad de San Carlos de Guatemala, Guatemala.

Institute of Nutrition of Central America and Panamá (INCAP) (1965) Informe Anual. Guatemala.

Inter-American Development Bank (1979) Nutrition and Socio-Economic Development of Latin America. Washington, DC.

Jul, Mogens (1978) "The Protein Situation in Developed Versus Developing Countries." In Adler-Nissen, Jens, Bj;yrn O. Eggum, Lars Munck, and Hans Sejr Olsen (eds.), Biochemical Aspects of New Protein Food, pp. 203–211. Oxford: Pergamon Press.

Montgomery, John D. (1977) "Food for Thought: On Appraising Nutrition Programs." Policy Sciences 8:

Plan Nacional de Salud 1978–1982 Ministerio de Salud Pública y Asistencia Social, Dirección General de Servicios de Salud, Guatemala.

Solien de González, N. L. (1964) Beliefs and Practices Concerning Medicine and Nutrition among Lower-Class Urban Guatemalans," American Journal of Public Health 54:

Urrutia, Juan José, Charles Teller, Victor Mejia Pivaral, Bertha Garcia, Marina Flores, Eileen Kennedy, Carlos Sequiera, and James E. Austin (1977) "Case Study: Guatemala." In Austin, James E. (ed.), Global Malnutrition and Cereal Fortification. Unpublished report to Agency for International Development, Contract AID/ta-C-1172, pp. 169–258.

Wise, Robert P. (1978) "Informe Preliminar del Resultado de la Encuesta del Programa Ampliado de Inmunizaciones, Totonicapán, Guatemala, Noviembre y Diciembre, 1977." Washington, DC: Offset, Pan American Health Organization. "The Case of Incaparina in Guatemala." (1980) Food and Nutrition Bulletin 2(2):3–8. "The Persistence of Poor Health in Guatemala: (1982) A Preventive Medical Perspective, Part I." Journal of Latin Community Health 1(1):71–79.

CHAPTER 14

Medical Modernization in Mexico: Paradigms, Labor Markets and the State

Julio Frenk

Discussed are the development of modern medical institutions in contemporary Mexico with a series of macrosocial changes. These are the expansion of State intervention in medical care, the labor market processes that eventually led to the appearance of medical unemployment, and the responses of the medical education system. It is expected that this kind of integrative analysis will help to understand the complex dynamics that characterize the health care patterns of developing societies.

Introduction

MEXICAN MEDICINE FACES TODAY A PRESSING PARADOX: while 14 million people, representing close to one-fifth of the population, lack access to medical services (Poder Ejecutivo Federal, 1984), it is believed that some 18,000 physicians are unemployed or underemployed (Frenk, 1985). This situation is not accidental; instead, it derives from the "model of medical development" (Foucault, 1976) that the country has followed. If the imbalances inherent in this model are to be corrected, it becomes necessary to examine its basic features in a broad historical light. What such an analysis reveals is the intricate interplay among three processes: the increasing involvement of the State in the organization of medical care, the quantitative and qualitative changes of the medical labor market, and the emergence of alternative paradigms about what modern medical care is, and how it becomes institutionalized by the medical education system. While Mexico's efforts to develop an "advanced" health system date back to colonial days, this chapter will focus on the period after 1958, when the contradictions among the three aforementioned processes have become most acute.

The Place of Traditional Medicine

At the time of the Spanish conquest in 1521, Mexico had a well-developed system of health care. It is doubtful that European medicine had at that time any therapeutic advantage over Indian practices. Nevertheless, the fact that these practices were an integral part of Indian religion and culture made their destruction by the Spaniards a necessary part of the cultural struggle that consolidated economic, political, and military domination (Mercer, 1984; Coheto-Martínez, 1984).

The medical conquest of ancient Mexico was never a complete process. Traditional beliefs and practices continued to play a crucial role during most of the colonial period. Even today, they shape most of the health care of the remaining ten million Indians and other rural inhabitants. Yet, the early and explicit attempts to neutralize traditional medicine have made it a less pervasive element in the contemporary health care arena of Mexico than of other Third World countries. Furthermore, it must be remembered that Mexico was the cradle of European medicine in the Western hemisphere. Indeed, it was there that the first medical course was taught, the first hospital built, and the first medical textbook printed. For these reasons, the central issue of medical modernization in

Mexico has not been the defeat or cooptation of traditional practice—though this is still an important problem and a point of controversy. For the bulk of health care, however, modernization has meant a succession of competing paradigms within European medicine. The rest of this chapter will focus on the adoption of one of those paradigms—namely, "scientific medicine"—and on the imbalances that such process has produced.

Early Institution-Building

The seeds of modern, scientific medicine were planted in Mexico around 1920. After more than one century of civil strife through the wars of Independence (1810–1821), Reform (1858–1867), and Revolution (1910–1920), conditions were ripe for an energetic effort at economic, cultural, and scientific reconstruction led by the postrevolutionary State. In 1924 the first specialized wards (for cardiology, gastroenterology, and urology) were created at the General Hospital of Mexico. During the 1940s, national specialty institutes were established in the fields of pediatrics, cardiology, and nutrition and internal medicine. In addition, the federal government created, in 1943, the Ministry of Sanitation and Public Assistance and the Mexican Institute of Social Security, which was to provide medical care to the blue-collar workers of the rapidly growing industrial plant. The institution-building efforts of the first half of the twentieth century set the stage for radically new form of conceiving, organizing, practicing, and teaching medicine. In this process, the State assumed the leading modernizing role, operating through the medical labor market and the medical education system.

The Modernizing Role of the State

The period from 1958 to 1967 witnessed an unparalleled transformation of the medical care system in Mexico through a very marked expansion of the participation of the public sector in the production of health services. As Donnangelo (1975) points out, the growth of State intervention in medical care has both a quantitative and a qualitative expression. The former involves an increase in the volume of services brought about by devoting more public resources to medical care and by extending the coverage of the population.

On the qualitative side, the expansion of State intervention usually entails a redefinition of the prevailing paradigms about medical practice. Compared to Kuhn's classical formulation (Kuhn, 1970), our usage of the term paradigm is broader, denoting, for the specific areas of medical care, an ideological model about the form, content, and organization of medical work, that is to say, a set of rules that prescribe, in a normative fashion, the ways in which human and material resources should be combined to produce ideal types of medical services. Medical care establishments represent a prime example of what Meyer and Rowan (1977) call "institutionalized organizations," which are subject to external normative prescriptions—for instance, through myths of rationality—about their legitimate structure and functions. The State is one of the basic sources of these prescriptions, as it represents a major agent for rationalization and modernization (Meyer, 1980).

In the late fifties and early sixties the new paradigm about medical care that started emerging in Mexico and that accompanied the expansion of State intervention was the paradigm of the what has been called "scientific medicine" (Berliner, 1975), as expressed in a highly rationalized mode of medical practice, one that is based on the division of medical work according to specific specialties, that finds its preferred space of action in the centralized structure of the hospital, and that fits the institutional framework of State-owned or State-financed organizations offering high levels of technological and administrative resources. Indeed, from 1958 to 1967 the Mexican State reoriented the basic definitions regarding the types of *sites* where medical care would be predominantly produced, the types of *activities* that would determine the character of medical work, and the types of institutional settings which would dominate the production of medical services.

First, with regard to the sites of health care, there was a definite shift from ambulatory to hospital practice. For instance, the number of medical care units with beds that belonged to the Mexican Institute of Social Security grew by 63 per cent in just the five years from 1959 to 1964, and the total number of beds actually doubled during the same period. In a parallel fashion, the Ministry of Sanitation and Public Assistance increased the number of its hospitals from 238 in 1959 to 731 in 1964. The emerging predominance of the hospital was epitomized by the construction of large medical centers that grouped several specialty hospitals (Frenk et al., 1980).

As far as the change in the dominant types of activities is concerned, there was a movement away from general and into specialty practice. As indicated earlier, this trend had started since the decade of the forties, when several semiautonomous specialty hospitals and institutes were founded. During the period of fast expansion of State intervention the role of specialization as the organizing principle of the production of medical services became consolidated. This process was reflected, for instance, in the creation of tertiary medical centers and in the growth of residency programs, which by the 1950s were present in almost all of the hospitals in Mexico City (Kumate et al., 1977:411). As a consequence, the ratio of generalists to specialists working for the Mexican Institute of Social Security went from 1.75 in 1961 to 0.93 in 1975 (Frenk et al., 1980).

Finally, the relative dominance of the various types of institutions that provide medical care also changed during the period we are considering. To begin with, the State became the major source of regulation and production in the market for medical services, overshadowing the private sector in terms of population covered and volume of services. And within the public sector itself the social security system began to acquire a central position at the expense of the public assistance institutions. This process deepened the class diversity of the Mexican health care system. Not only did private services remain reserved for the privileged few that could afford them, but, in addition, the public sector became divided into a two-class system: social security institutions with large resources to take care of blue- and white-collar workers mostly in urban areas, versus public assistance organizations responsible, with considerably less resources, for the health of the rural population and the urban poor (Soberón and Narro, 1984).

Why did the social security system become the motor of State intervention in medical care? An important factor seems to have been the series of 740 strikes that affected the country in 1958 (Mesa-Lago, 1978). As a response to these strikes, the State extended social benefits, including medical care. Indeed, "(s)ocial security concessions were instruments used to restore social peace. . ." (Mesa-Lago, 1978:218). Just as public assistance represented a means for legitimizing the regime that emerged from the Mexican Revolution, so did social security constitute the organized response of the State to the changing realities of urbanization and industrialization, including the need for a healthy and productive labor force. Furthermore, the fact that the social security system covered blue and white collar workers made it particularly compatible with the corporatist structure of interest representation that prevails in Mexico (Schmitter, 1979; Pereyra, 1979). Because of these factors and of its state protected financing, the social security system in Mexico has been able to provide the administrative and technical resources necessary for the institutionalization of scientific medicine in Mexico.

The Response of the Medical Education System

The rapid expansion of State intervention in medical care that took place from 1958 to 1967 introduced two changes in the medical labor market: a) a quantitative increase in the manpower requirements of the medical care system and b) a qualitative reorientation in the dominant forms of medical work and therefore in the types of skills that physicians were expected to master. The medical education system was able to respond adequately to the latter but not to the former.

On the qualitative front, a major reform of medical education revised the curricular structure so as to better adapt it to the shift towards specialty and hospital practice. Prior to this reform, most medical schools in Mexico maintained a curriculum whose clinical portion (following two years of basic sciences) was still very much influenced by the French tradition, with three years of general clinical instruction that was mostly based on the rather unspecialized distinction between internal (i.e., medical) and external (i.e., surgical) phenomena. The needs for practical training of medical students were satisfied, during the sixth year, by a "practicum." This was only a part-time activity to be discharged by working a few hours in some hospitals after attending formal lectures and being on duty some occasional nights every week. In a parallel fashion, students might learn directly from the practice of medicine by becoming informal assistants to established physicians. All this was changed in 1960, when the National University of Mexico formally approved a new curriculum for the School of Medicine, which introduced an organization of clinical courses based on the specialized study of each organ or system. The sixth year of this new curriculum was occupied entirely by an internship, whereby students were required, for the first time, to devote one year to full-time activities in a hospital before obtaining their medical degrees (Kumate et al., 1977).

The internship provided future physicians with the practical skills that would allow them to work in hospital settings. Quantitatively, it also represented a means to satisfy part of the new manpower requirements brought about by the expansion in State production of medical services. This role of the internship was particularly important, as it served to compensate, in the short run, the lack of a commensurate growth of the supply of graduate physicians (Frenk et al., 1983). For instance, enrollment at the School of Medicine of the National University of Mexico remained practically constant between 1958 and 1967 (Oficina de Planeación y Programación, 1978). Further, from 1961 to 1965 no new schools of medicine were opened, and from 1966 to 1970 only four such schools started functioning (Subsecretaría de Planeación, 1977).

The Appearance of Medical Unemployment

Starting in 1967, and even more so since the early 1970, the quantitative relationship between the medical education and the medical care systems assumed almost the mirror image of the previous decade. While the growth of the health care sector slowed down and even diminished in certain aspects, the medical education system experienced an explosive expansion. Thus, a stagnant public investment in medical care led to a reduction in the rate of growth of services produced and of number of beds, both in the Mexican Institute of Social Security and the Ministry of Sanitation and Public Assistance. For example, the number of beds belonging to the Institute grew from 1959 to 1967 at an annual rate of 12 per cent, compared to only 4 per cent between 1967 and 1976. Likewise, from 1959 to 1967 the production of ambulatory visits increased at an annual rate of 9 per cent and the number of hospital admissions at a rate of 15 per cent. From 1967 to 1976 the corresponding figures were 5 and 7 per cent, respectively (Frenk et al., 1980).

At the same time, the system of medical education started growing through two processes: first the expansion of enrollment in the existing schools and then the creation of a large number of new schools. In just four years, total student enrollment in the country increased by 20,000, as it jumped from 20,127 in 1967 to 41,675 in 1971–72 (Rodríguez, 1974). By 1977 one source estimated that there were 80,396 medical students in Mexico (Dirección General de Servicios Coordinados de Salud Pública en los Estados, 1978). The number of medical schools doubled from 26 in 1970 to 54 in 1980 (Hernández-Chávez, 1982:161–164).

The common determinant of both the slowdown in the health care sector and the growth of the medical education system appears to have been the economic crisis that affected the country in the 1970s. On the one hand, the rate of growth of federal spending for social programs, including medical care, was reduced; on the other, the Mexican government followed a policy of expanding the middle and higher educational systems (Fuentes and Noriega, 1979). While this was never explicitly acknowledged by government officials, it is not unreasonable to presume that such a policy was carried out in order to absorb part of the young population which, given the economic conditions of the country, could not find a job. An additional factor that might in part explain the growth of higher education refers to political demands by the middle classes for easier access to what they perceive as one of the most legitimate channels of upward mobility. In any event, it is clear that the institutions of middle and higher education have added to their traditional functions the role of postponing pressures on the general labor market. One important consequence of this process, however, has been the appearance of unemployment among university graduates. In the case of medicine, there were approximately 8,000 graduates in 1978. Yet only 1,800 positions for residency were available, and a reliable source estimated that the private and the public sectors combined could absorb no more than 3,000 new physicians per year (Rivero, 1978). This would mean that approximately forty per cent of the graduates were faced with the prospect of becoming underemployed or unemployed after six years of medical studies. As indicated at the beginning of this paper, current estimates place the total of unemployed or underemployed physicians at 18,000 though the exact figure is not known.

Primary Health Care: An Emerging Paradigm?

The coexistence of doctors without jobs and people without doctors has brought forth the limitations of the prevailing paradigm based on specialty and hospital care. The end of the seventies seems to have marked a fundamental shift in health care policy. Concepts such as universal access, right to health care, primary care, and community participation define the new discourse of modernity in the health arena.

Starting in 1979, when the resources generated by the oil boom could have sustained the continued growth of specialty hospitals, two large-scale innovative programs were launched to extend basic health care coverage. The first one was a "social solidarity" program, run by the Mexican Institute of Social Security, to care for the uninsured rural population. As a result of this effort, over 3,000 rural medical units and 1,600 beds in rural general hospitals were built, with a coverage of 11 million people (Poder Ejecutivo Federal, 1984). The second program, which began in 1981, developed a modern network of 255 health centers for over 4 million slum dwellers of the large cities.

Both of these programs opened new employment opportunities for physicians who were willing to practice general or family medicine in rural and periurban areas. At the same time, there was a reduction in the growth of medical schools, reflecting that they had reached saturation levels in the recent past and also that a prosperous economy offered a greater diversity of options to the young. Despite these favorable developments, the expansion of medical school enrollments that had taken place during the previous decade remained, so that the supply of physicians continued to exceed the demand.

With the severe economic crisis that began in 1982, there was a large risk that the State might revert to the usual response of cutting social programs. Instead, the new administration that came into power on December of 1982 declared that health care was one of its top priorities, since it is precisely in times of economic crisis that the majority of the population can least afford cuts in social programs. The new elements of medical modernization in Mexico include a constitutional amendment recognizing the right to health care; the formulation of a National Health Program that will rationalize activities; an energetic attempt to decentralize the system so that state governments may run their health programs with greater responsiveness to local needs; the integration of a National Health System that will provide overall coordination; and an ambitious goal of finally extending health care coverage to all the population.

Conclusion

The foregoing historical analysis has revealed a deep and rich connection linking medical modernization with transformations in the conditions of the medical labor market and also, ultimately, with broader processes of social and economic development. It would be interesting to investigate whether the relationships discussed here also hold in other countries. Indeed, it seems necessary to pursue integrative studies that connect the macrosocial phenomena of State intervention in medical care, medical labor markets, and professionalization to specific forms of organization of medical practice and medical education. Analyses of this kind would greatly advance the elaboration of a comparative theory of medical care that would allow a better understanding of the intricate patterns of health care in the world today.

Parts of this paper are reprinted from Education Medica y Salud, Vol. 18, No. 4 (1984) pp. 329–343 by permission of the author and publisher.

References

Berliner, Howard S. (1975) "A larger perspective on the Flexner Report." International Journal of Health Services 5:573–91.

Coheto-Martínez, Cándido V. (1984) "Problemática de salud en las áreas de población indígena y medicina tradicional." ("Health problems in areas with Indian population and traditional medicine"). Paper presented at the II Interamerican Conference on Health Education. Mexico City, November, 1984.

Dirección General de Servicios Coordinados de Salud Pública en los Estados (1978) "Análisis sobre el ejercicio de la medicina en

México y sus proyecciones." ("Analysis and projections of the practice of medicine in Mexico"). Unpublished document.

Foucault, Michel (1976) "La crisis de la medicina o la crisis de la antimedicina." ("The crisis of medicine or the crisis of antimedicine"). Educación Médica y Salud 10:152–70.

Frenk, Julio (1985) "Career preferences under conditions of medical unemployment: The case of interns in Mexico." Medical Care, in press.

Frenk, Julio, Héctor Hernándes-Llamas and Lourdes Alvarez-Klein (1980) "El mercado de trabajo médico. II. Evolución histórica en México." (The medical labor market. II. Historical evolution in Mexico"). Gaceta Médica de México 116:265–84.

"Análisis histórico del internado rotatorio de pregrado en México." (1983) ("Historical analysis of the rotating undergraduate internship in Mexico"). Gaceta Médica de México 119:87–96.

Fuentes, Olac and M. Noriega (1979) "La política educativa del Estado mexicano a través del financiamiento federal 1959–1976." ("The educational policy of the Mexican State, through federal financing. 1959–1976"). Unpublished document.

Hernández-Chávez, Abel (1982) Estado Actual de la Educación Médica en México. (Current State of Medical Education in Mexico). México, D. F.: Asociación Mexicana de Facultades y Escuelas de Medicina.

Kuhn, Thomas S. (1970) The Structure of Scientific Revolutions. (Second Edition). Chicago: University of Chicago Press.

Kumate, Jesús, Luis Cañedo and Oscar Pedrotta (1977) La Salud de los Mexicanos y la Medicina en México. (The Health of Mexicans and Medicine in Mexico). México, D. F.: Editorial de El Colegio Nacional.

Mercer, Hugo (1984) "Hospitales y práctica médica en la ciudad de México." ("Hospitals and medical practice in Mexico City"). Estudios Sociológicos 2:335–49.

Mesa-Lago, Carmelo (1978) Social Security in Latin America: Pressure Groups, Stratification, and Inequality. Pittsburgh: University of Pittsburgh Press.

Meyer, John W. (1980) "The World polity and the authority of the nation-state." Pp. 109–37 in Albert Bergesen (ed.), Studies of the Modern World-System. New York: Academic Press.

Meyer, John W. and Brian Rowan (1977) "Institutionalized organizations: Formal structure as myth and ceremony." American Journal of Sociology 83:340–63.

Oficina de Planeación y Programación (1978) Unpublished data on enrollments at the National Autonomous University of Mexico.

Pereyra, Carlos (1979) "Estado y sociedad." ("State and society"). Pp. 289–305 in Pablo González-Casanova and Enrique Florescano (eds.), México, Hoy. (Mexico Today). México, D. F.: Siglo Veintiuno Editores.

Poder Ejecutivo Federal (1984) Programa Nacional de Salud 1984–1988. (National Health Program 1984–1988). México, D. F. Secretaría de Salubridad y Asistencia.

Rivero, Octavio (1978) "Situación actual de la enseñanza de la medicina." ("Current situation of medical education"). Unpublished document.

Rodríguez, María Isabel (1974) "El estudiante de medicina—su distribución en las Américas, 1971–1972." ("The medical student—his distribution in the America, 1971–1972"). Educación Médica y Salud 8:360–89.

Schmitter, Philippe C. (1979) "Still the century of corporatism?" Pp. 7–52 in Philippe C. Schmitter and Gerhard Lehmbruch (eds.), Trends Toward Corporatist Intermediation. Beverly Hills and London: Sage.

Soberón, Guillermo and José Narro (1984) "Equity and health care in Latin America: Principles and dilemmas." Paper presented at the Conference on Health Policy, Ethics and Human Values: An International Dialogue. Athens, Greece.

Subsecretaría de Planeación (1977) Educación de Pregrado en Medicina y Enfermería. (Undergraduate Education in Medicine and Nursing). México, D. F.: Secretaría de Salubridad y Asistencia.

Political Ideology, Armed Conflict and Modern Health Care Delivery

CHAPTER 15

Cuban Health Care:
A Study in Consumer Control

Peter Orris

This chapter is a description of user participation in the
Cuban health care system. It considers: citizen involvement in planning, concurrent review and execution.

Introduction

ON JULY 26, 1953, FIDEL CASTRO, A YOUNG LAWYER, AND A
group primarily composed of students attacked the Monceda
Military Barracks in Santiago de Cuba, ushering in a new era
of struggle against the Batista Military dictatorship.

The attack was a failure and those not killed were jailed, yet
this event set the stage for the coming revolution. The revolutionary struggle conducted by Castro with broad support
amongst the peasants and workers of Cuba was successful on
January 1, 1959. These young revolutionaries then began to
initiate wide ranging social programs, chief among which was
the development of a comprehensive national health care
system paid for by the government.

Health Care:

Cuba's health conditions were not bad prior to the revolution when compared with the health standards of Latin America as a whole. By 1959, the country had 6,300 physicians, many of whom had been trained in the United States. This represented a physician-patient ratio of one doctor per thousand population, a rather impressive figure for Latin America. The difficulty hidden by this figure, however, is the fact that 63% of these physicians were in Havana. The others were in the few other large cities with almost none in the rural areas. (Orris, 1970)

Morbidity and mortality rates for most diseases were lower in Cuba than for other countries in Latin America. Yet the situation was far from optimal, especially in the areas of the controllable infectious diseases. The data available on Cuba disease rates prior to 1961 is incomplete and must be considered underestimated since there was no systematic collection for the country. In addition, little attention was paid to the rural population during this period. (Orris, 1970)

A qualitative look at the problem is revealed when the story of the problem of the peasants in Oriente Province in the mountains of the Sierra Maestra is recounted. In order to receive health care, a peasant in the hills had to travel up to two days on horseback or by foot to reach the southern coast of Cuba. There the patient would light a fire on a bluff overlooking the ocean and wait for a boat to pass. Hopefully, that boat would transport him/her to Santiago where the nearest hospital was located. Clearly, only the sickest person would undertake this journey and many died along the way. A graveyard on a bluff outside the small village of Ochuhal on the coast is grim testimony of these facts. If the peasant died at home or along the way, he/she never made it into the national health statistics.

Around the turn of the century, Spanish ethnic groups in Cuba laid the basis for prepaid insurance organizations called "Mutualistas." By 1950 those prepaid health insurance organizations became very popular in urban areas, yet the premium charged the user was higher than most Cuban workers could afford, and was not designed to cover all costs of medical care. (Danielson, 1970)

Government activities in health care were limited. It operated hospitals, maternity clinics, dental clinics, and some first aid stations. These once again were centered in the cities and quality was irregular because of administrative blunders and graft. A certain amount of preventive medicine was also practiced by the government. Vaccinations were given in the face of epidemics, and other services were available on a fee-for-service basis. The World Health Organization's report of 1964 indicates that these efforts prior to 1959 in Cuba were inadequate. (WHO, 1964)

With the success of the rebellion in 1959, the new leadership of the country was faced with the immense task of constructing a new governmental structure reflecting their ideals. They conceptualized the principles upon which they based their health care system as follows:

1. Integration at each level of the system of preventive and curative medicine.
2. Centralization of policy in the Ministry of Public Health at a national level, with administrative decisions handled as locally as possible.
3. Emphasis was placed on the previously underserved areas which were primarily rural.
4. Integral participation of the population in the work of the health system.
5. Planning for health care within the general direction and policy of the government as a whole.
6. Increased attention to research with intimate coordination between the national research institutes and those institutions providing health care to the population.
7. Collective work at all levels.
8. Creating and centralizing all health activities into a

single branch of government, the Ministry of Public Health (MinSaP.)

9. Placing emphasis on maternal and child health.
10. Opening medical education to all, regardless of race, sex, or economic position. (Orris, 1981)

The health care of the population became a national priority of the new government. By 1982, 397 urban polyclinics were operating and 142 dental clinics. The total number of hospitals in Cuba has increased from 57 in 1959 to 256 in 1981. The number of beds has gone from 28,536 to 47,327. One rural hospital was operated in 1959 in the guerilla zone with 10 beds while today there are 52 rural hospitals. Laboratories of hygiene and microbiology now number 30, fourteen with emphasis on the industrial environment, where none existed in 1959. There are also now 21 blood banks on the island. (Ministerio Salude Publica, 1982)

As is suggested by the steady increase in services, government expenditures on health care have risen from $3.5 per capita in 1959 to $19.9 in 1969 and comprises over 15% of the Gross National Product today. (Ubell, 1983:1468) Physician visits, which numbered 5.0 per inhabitant in 1981 had increased from 3.0 in 1967. Institutionalized births are now practically universal, as opposed to 1959 when it was estimated only 50% of babies were born in hospitals. There has been a concomitant marked decrease in infant mortality over this period, from 39.5 in 1967 to 17.3 in 1982. (Orris, 1970:86, Ubell, 1983)

The Health Area is the basic geographical unit of the public health system. These areas are organized on the basis of population and accessibility of facilities. In urban settings 25,000 to 35,000 people are covered by each area. In certain rural areas, where travel is especially difficult and time between home and health facility lengthy, as few as 7,500 people may be included in the health area.

Each urban Health Area is serviced by a polyclinic. The polyclinic is supervised by a Director, with a Technical Committee and a Consumer Health Commission. Polyclinic personnel include statisticians. administrators, dental workers, and a general practitioner or internist for each sector of approximately 2,000 inhabitants; an obstetrician and pediatrician for every two sectors; and two nurses for each sector. Also responsible to the Director of the polyclinic are the various pharmacies in the health area. (Orris, 1970)

The counterpart of the urban polyclinic is the rural hospital in rural areas. These hospitals have smaller staffs in the clinical areas because their population base is smaller. Inpatient and outpatient medical care for simple problems, hygienic services, contagious disease control, well-baby care and prenatal counseling, statistical collection and health education are all offered. Factories with over 1,000 workers have a doctor and a nurse stationed at the plant. If the plant is judged particularly dangerous, it has a physician for over 500 workers. This service provides first aid, outpatient acute care for common problems, and the personnel are involved in health promotion and control of hazards in the plant.

Each local political division, the municipality, has between five and nine health areas in it. There is a municipal hospital offering most specialties including traumatology, surgery, internal medicine, dermatology and psychiatry on an inpatient and outpatient basis. In addition, old-age homes are administered at this level as are specialty dental clinics, preventive services, public health laboratories and blood banks coordinated by the central Municipal health ministry office. The municipal health system is governed by the twin bodies of the Health Commission and Technical Committee, which are directly responsible to the municipal legislature, the "Poder Popular" and Provincial health ministry leadership.

In Cuba's 14 Provinces, all specialty services of university medical centers are available. Health Planning departments and specialized public health laboratories exist at this level as well. The provincial Poder Popular and the national health ministry have oversight and policy control of the provincial health activities.

National research institutes have been organized, responsible directly to the public health ministry. Of these, the Cardiovascular Institute is one of the largest and fastest growing. This institute has the latest in electronic equipment including mobile intensive care units, cardiac care units, cardiac catheterization equipment and capabilities for open heart surgery.

Another aspect of the Institute's work is especially interesting in light of the recent developments in the field of cardiovascular epidemiology. Since the people of Cuba are organized on a block by block basis in voluntary organizations, including Committees for the Defense of the Revolution (CDR), Federation of Cuban Women (FMC), and the Association of Small Farmers (ANAP), the possibility for accurate prospective studies of chronic disease and risk factors is evident. The CDR's functions include guarding and protecting the revolution's property against saboteurs, study circles on political themes, as well as periodic "Days of Solidarity" with other peoples of the world. Local CDR's also organize aid for the educational facilities in the area, and stimulate popular participation in the government.

Some members of the local CDR's aid officials in the maintenance of a clean neighborhood, and other tasks involved in keeping the edifices of the area operating and in good condition. Around each city and town there are fields that the CDR's maintain by voluntary labor on Sundays, with the produce going directly to the government. Committees recruit for the local militia, and organize sports activities, plays and festivals. (Sarmiento, 1969) With the active participation of these organizations, studies are being planned to identify environmental risk factors and outcomes of therapy.

Citizen Involvement in the Health System

Planning

In Cuba there is a large degree of citizen involvement in the health care system. The primary vehicles created for the participation of citizens in the planning of health policy is through health commissions. These health commissions were organized at every level of the ministry of health in the early 1960's. The membership includes one representative from each ministry concerned with living conditions, such as the Committees for the Defense of the Revolution (CDR), Federation of Cuban Women (FMC), Association of Small Farmers (ANAP) and Confederation of Cuban Trade Unions (CTC). The Communist Party (PCC), the Young Communist League (UJC), and the personnel of the Ministry of Public Health also attend the meetings.

The medical input on these commissions is quite important. Physicians are charged with the responsibility of outlining the problems of health and indicating possible preventive steps to be taken. This in essence placed the primary power inside the commission within the sphere of the physicians in that they "set the agenda." The other groups performed more of a consultative task. The paramount responsibility of these health commissions therefore is to prepare the long and short range tasks and goals for the Ministry of Health.

Evaluation:

These are many ways of handling patient complaints in Cuba. They are essentially the same in both urban and rural areas. The health care system is able to assess patient satisfaction prior to, during, or following an episode of health care. A dissatisfied recipient of a health service in Cuba can complain to the director of the facility involved. In Havana at the Polyclinic Reina, the director reported that he received several of these complaints a month and that most are settled within the polyclinic. The most common complaint reported was verbal insensitivity by staff members. The most common remedy was a talk between the staff member and the director about the incident. If this did not suffice, a meeting was set up between the complainant, the staff member, and the director.

This type of complaint procedure was reported by all the primary and many of the referral facilities visited. The average

rate appeared to be a few a month with the exception of the
rural hospitals. There were fewer patients, and consequently a
lower number of complaints in the rural facilities.

Complaints could also be made to any staff member. Specific staff members, "advanced workers," were required to be
alert to patient problems and complaints. They were to actively seek the complaints or comments about the services
from patients. They solicited these from patients during waiting periods or other non-treatment times at the center. These
were by and large verbal communications.

If a patient was having an argument with a staff member of
the polyclinic, these specified staff members were to side with
the patient and aid in the resolution of the conflict to the
satisfaction of the patient. The system seems to be an effort to
incorporate workers who will act, part time, as what U.S.
health professionals call "patient advocates." In the final resolution it may be determined that the patient was not correct,
but he/she had received the support of someone he/she visu-
alized as part of the system during the process of the conflict.

At the primary level outside of the health facility itself, a
complaint about the services at a primary or referral unit can
be made by any citizen to a member of the Communist Party,
Young Communist League, Poder Popular representative, or
the neighborhood health activist of the CDR, FMC, or ANAP.

If the complainant was not satisfied with either the resolution within the facility or with an advocate from outside the
Health Ministry, the individual could carry the complaint in
person or writing to the Municipal Pader Popular, Communist
Party, or Health Ministry personnel. This process can also be
repeated through the provincial and national levels.

The final method available to a citizen was to write or see
Fidel Castro. Many Cubans did just that, and bypassed all the
other structures. Castro has responded to such appeals and
has gone to local areas in Cuba to try to redress a grievance
that a citizen had addressed to him. The popular belief was
that this was a common occurrence and therefore a viable

option for the individual. The differences in procedures between the facilities visited by the author all centered around lowering the threshold of complaints, and insuring the regular collection of comments from patients.

Implementation:

The use of non-professional citizens in the execution of health tasks is a major part of the programs of the Ministry of health. Citizens are involved primarily in health education as well as disease prevention on a day-to-day basis.

There have been a series of national citizen campaigns attacking some of the serious health problems of the island. For example, the Anti-Polio Vaccination Campaigns by the CDR and the Health Ministry of 1962 through 1966. Polio epidemics occurred in Cuba in 1942, 1946, 1952 and 1955. These epidemics saw the mortality rate per 100,000 inhabitants rise to between 4.4 and 10 with over 492 cases in 1952 and 267 in 1959. Between the years 1959 and 1961, the mortality rate remained at a high of between 4 and 5 with between 200 to 350 cases a year. (Sarmiento, 1969)

CDR's were responsible for organizing the vaccination of children. The vaccine used was the Sabin oral vaccine acquired from the USSR in candy form. Individuals from the CDR block committees made a thorough search in the area to insure that every child was covered. Not one case of polio has been found in Cuba since 1964. (Ministerio DeSalud Publica, 1982)

The basic unit for the implementation of the day to day activities of the health ministry is the individual in the CDR local block committee who is responsible for health work called "responsable de Salud." This person coordinates the activities in the health area of the local committee members, and the technical personnel of the polyclinic. Local health assemblies are organized by these people as educational forums for people in the area to learn about health topics. Organizing the neighborhood to maintain sanitary conditions in the area is also a job of the health representative. The block responsable de Salud is the link between the citizen and the health system.

Problems of the Health Care System
After 20 Years of Growth

The Ministry of Health was established in 1963. In 1974 most of the construction of new health facilities that had been projected was either finished or in progress. The shortage of health personnel was largely a problem of the past. Medical students were now able to specialize in the full range of subspecialities, and many types that were previously only available through study abroad were being given in Cuba.

The infectious disease killers of children and the poor of pre-revolutionary Cuba had been eradicated or significantly reduced. In the 1970's the health picture of the population was vastly improved, with the new challenges facing the health ministry—those posed by chronic diseases. All these accomplishments were extraordinary, but not enough.

In 1974, the leadership of the Ministry of Public Health set out to assess the satisfaction of the people with the system. A national study group made up of 12 physicians of all major specialties and those people responsible for the health programs of the major voluntary peoples organizations, brought out a report a year later. The report noted, to the surprise of the Health Ministry, that many of their goals were not being met.

As one example, though the system set as its goal the emphasis on primary health care at polyclinics, people were still utilizing the emergency rooms of large city hospitals as their first access to health care. This created fragmented health care delivery and difficulty in accurate, comprehensive record keeping. Also, it overtaxed emergency rooms with non-emergent cases. One hospital in Havana, Calixto Garcia, was seeing almost 1,000 patients a day with only one out of 10 having urgent problems. Part of the reason for this utilization pattern were old ideas created prior to 1959 when the only good care available was to be had at large hospitals. Further, certain approaches of the Ministry reinforced this thinking. For example, in order to eradicate gastroenteritis as a childhood killer, the health ministry advised Cuban citizens to take their children to a hospital at the first sign of significant diarrhea. Women who were to give birth were told that they should have their children in a hospital. Also, the great emigration of doctors to the U.S. in the early 1060's, the good clinicians were needed to train new physicians, which at that time was done almost entirely in the large hospitals with medical school affiliations. This created a shortage of dedicated superior clinicians in polyclinics. Finally, most polyclinics were not open after working hours, leaving working Cubans with no choice but to seek the hospital emergency room.

The feedback or assessment of citizen satisfaction with the health system underwent the most devastating re-evaluation by the Cubans. The original system conceived of in 1963 was thought at the time and for the next decade to be an effective method of assessing satisfaction and efficient use of the system. Following the work of the national commission in 1976, this view was shattered. The Ministry made its findings known and engaged in strenuous activity to correct the problems. The first and most obvious failure of the original system was apparent in the fact that simple complaints such as long waits and poor scheduling of consultation hours were not heard or heeded by the system at the local or regional level. A national commission was necessary to discover these problems. Clearly, if a feedback system was operable, at least some local areas would have known about these problems and projected local solutions. This did not occur.

Possible explanations for this situation lay in a number of areas. Initially, the Cuban Health Ministry had the vast task of creating resources to service the population. The construction of new facilities and provision of new health personnel consumed much time, but further provided a convenient rationale on the part of the providers that all the problems of local communities lay in the scarcity of resources and not in poor organization. Secondly, the population never had any of these health resources available before. A population that never was exposed to health centers in the past, cannot be expected to use such centers efficiently until it acquires some experience in its use. The Health Ministry's policy emphasis was on outpatient care, and yet the practical advice to use inpatient hospital services, confused the public as to the proper use of the facilities.

Cuba's health commissions were structurally, though unintentionally designed to filter out criticisms, not collect them. They were made up of the most active community residents who were intimately involved on a daily basis with the functioning of the health system. These citizens were the most committed to the revolution and the tasks of the Ministry. This gave them a built-in identification with the providers of the health service and not with its users. Many criticisms of the functioning of the system were probably stifled even prior to their being presented to the health professionals by the community health activist. The activists, by their very involvement in the health tasks of the Ministry, had a stake in rationalizing its shortcomings.

Approaches to the Solution of These Problems

In 1976 the Ministry of Public Health projected a new approach to the involvement of the health system in the community. This new approach was based on six objectives designed to strengthen the founding principles of Cuba's health care system formulated in 1963. They were directed at primary care given in urban polyclinics and rural hospitals. These objectives were:

1. The health care services were to be integrated. The activities of the primary care institution in the areas of preventive and curative medicine now were to be inte-

grated with concerns for the individual and community psychological and social conditions. Increased attention was to be placed on the smallest division of the polyclinic areas, the sector.

2. With the increasing specialization of the primary care staff, a need for inter-sector communication was a necessity. The physicians and other health workers in the polyclinic were to have regular meetings to coordinate their work within the area. These meetings were to cross specialty and job category lines with additional meetings planned in each area of specialty. Physicians were also to achieve greater interaction with the regional hospitals and other secondary facilities in their area.

3. Continuity of care was another area in need of strengthening. With the new policy, patients from each sector would see the same physician and nurse in their homes as they did on each visit to the polyclinic. These health professionals would follow the patients when they needed hospitalization as well. Physicians were to work with inpatient hospital staff to improve care during hospitalization and facilitate the recovery after discharge.

4. To eliminate the problem of perceiving polyclinic staffs as individuals to be consulted only when sick, physicians and nurses in each sector were to spend each afternoon visiting homes of chronically ill patients. These visits were to be planned on a regular basis to take care of prescription and treatment needs of diabetic, cardiac and other chronic patients. This would provide physicians with needed insights into the lifestyle of the patients so important for the care of the chronically ill.

5. Collective work was another area stressed in this new approach. This had been an objective of the ministry since 1963, but often had not been structurally incorporated in the day-to-day operations. This structural lack often led to physician domination of the health team and little contact between specialties. The new approach mandated multiple interdisciplinary conferences on theoretical and practical topics as well as the inclusion of

nurses and sanitary workers into the daily functioning of the primary care physicians. A primary care team of physicians was designated in each sector, including the internist, pediatrician, obstetrician, and gynecology physicians. This group was to meet and plan programs daily with nurses and other health workers in the sector.

6. Finally, the new approach mandated that the health workers in the sector meet regularly with local block committees and health volunteers of the Committees for the Defense of the Revolution. These meetings were small, allowing all present to speak and question the activities of the health workers. The conception here was to permit feedback as to the services of the health system.

The creation of the elected assemblies of the Poder Popular in 1976 and 1977, strengthen the consumer review and control of the health system. At each level of the legislative structure of the Poder Popular, a representative chaired the health commissions, with budgetary and policy control. The long term effects of these changes are not yet known. The need for them and the method of their implementation should be of great interest to all health planners.

References

Danielson, Ross (1970) Cuban Medicine, Transaction Press, New Jersey

Ministerio DeSalud Publica (1982) Informe Anual, Havana, Cuba

Orris, Peter (1970) The Role of the Consumer in the Cuban National Health System, Yale University School of Public Health

Orris, Peter (1981) The Sociology of Health and Medical Care: Citizens Involvement in Cuba 1959–1980, Red Feather Institute for Advanced Studies in Sociology

Sarmiento, O. V. (1969) Los CDR LaVacunacion Antipolio y el Tiempo Libre, Committees for the Defense of the Revolution

Sarmiento, O. V. (1969) International Conference on Community Development Alger, Algeria, March 4 (U.N.)

World Health Organization (1964) Third Report on the World Health Situation, Geneva, Switzerland.

CHAPTER 16

Community Participation and Politics in Malaria Control Activities in Nicaragua

Richard M. Garfield

In many areas of the world malaria has made a comeback as the usual methods to control the disease have become less effective. Pesticide sprays no longer bring the rapid and dramatic results which they showed when introduced after World War II. Innovative efforts more recently have focused on the use of community residents in affected areas to improve the environment, improve malaria diagnosis, and use medicines to prevent and cure the disease. This chapter details the largest experiment in preventing malaria via mass drug administration ever attempted. This effort occurred in Nicaragua in 1981. As is detailed below, the malaria campaign was a unique organizing effort which brought many results besides the short term prevention of malaria cases.

Introduction

MALARIA RESURGENCE HAS BEEN A PROBLEM ON FOUR continents since the early 1960's (U.S. G.A.O., 1982). Malaria is an infectious disease caused by the *Plasmodium* protozoa and transmitted from one person to another by the Anopheles mosquito. The *Plasmodium* parasite invades red blood cells, destroying them and causing a wide variety of symptoms including severe intermittent fevers, chills, body aches, and weakness. (Bruce-Chwatt; 1980).

While many possible methods exist to control the disease, few have actually been effective. Which methods will be effective in a particular area may depend on the local ecology, customs and politics. In many areas, community participation may be essential to reducing the malaria burden. It has not yet been fully established for which activities and in which areas community involvement will be key. More complex yet is to determine how to motivate community members to take part in anti-malarial efforts and learn about the disease, its prevention, and its cure.

Since history was first recorded, malaria has been considered the most common of the serious diseases. (Harrison; 1978). Large scale attacks on the disease after World War II with DDT sprays and improved anti-malarial drugs led to the hope that the disease would soon be eradicated. Indeed, for about a decade the number of cases found in most countries dropped rapidly. Since the early 1970's, however, the number of cases has mushroomed in what was finally recognized by the World Health Organization in 1976 as a resurgence of the disease. Tens of millions of people now contract the disease annually. In Africa alone one million children die of malaria each year.

The former chief of planning for malaria eradication at the World Health Organization wrote that, "The present resurgence of malaria poses a major threat to world health far greater than that which prompted the WHO eradication program of the 1950's" (Farid, 1980:1). Reasons for the resurgence include increasing resistance of the *Anopheles* mosquito to pesticides, increasing resistance of the *Plasmodium* protozoa to conventional drug therapy, decreased national and international funding, and the pressure of other competing health needs (Najera, 1979). Nonetheless, Farid argues that "the main reasons for the failure [of malaria eradication] have to be sought in the soft sciences—human behavior, politics, economics." Further, while most of the current research in malaria is oriented toward developing an immunizing vaccine and more effective antimalarial drugs, he admits that "we cannot expect to conquer malaria, a disease rooted in the physical and socioeconomic environment of tropical areas, by a miraculous vaccine, drug, or insecticide. Such scientific tools will be of great value, but their proper use will depend on other factors closely related to human ecology in its broadest sense." (Farid, 1980:8).

Before 1948 (when the pesticide DDT was first popularized) malaria was present in 39% of the total areas of the Americas, putting 36% of the population at risk for the disease (Garcia, 1972). In Central America malaria incidence has varied widely from year to year. During the first half of this century, it was the most frequent diagnosis and most common cause for hospitalization in the region. The "vicious cycle of malaria" is a high correlation between malaria and poverty, ignorance, illiteracy, and social deprivation. "Not only has malaria contributed more than its share to the human burden of poverty and ill health, but the syndrome of underdevelopment acts in numerous ways to foster the spread and to hinder the control of malaria" (Wessen, 1972:659). The control of malaria is thus thought to contribute to social and economic development; the way such control is achieved may influence developmental effects.

Control Methods

To reduce or eliminate the occurrence of the disease, many actions may be employed to 'break the chain' of transmission. First, contact between man and mosquito can be reduced. This can often be effected through sleeping under mosquito netting, using repellents, or avoiding the out-of-doors at night when mosquitoes bite. The reduction of the mosquito population is a more effective and sure means to reduce man-mosquito contact. Mosquitoes can be eliminated by destroying the places where they breed through changing water use patterns, killing the mosquito larvae before they hatch with oils or chemicals, introducing biological predators into the larval environment, or killing hatched adults with pesticide sprays. It must be remembered, though, that mosquitoes are only one link in the chain of this disease. Reduction of the number of cases of malaria in the human population will reduce the chance that mosquitoes can contract and transmit the disease. Earlier diagnosis and treatment will reduce the reservoir of infection among people. The optimal strategy will vary from country to country depending on the types and amounts of mosquitoes present, the degree of resistance to drugs and pesticides, the cultural and social habits of the population, and the economic structure of the country. These factors are all mediated by the potential and approach to community participation and popular education employed.

Malarial communities are usually poor. If community residents do not perceive the problem as their 'helpers' do, disagree with the values and behavior they display, find social contacts with them difficult or unrewarding, they are not likely to be motivated. (WHO; 1984). If they see one government official encourage community participation in health programs while another tries to destroy a newly established peasants' union, they may be suspicious about the authorities' motives and cynical about the potential benefit to them. (ECLA; 1973). These disincentives to participation may manifest themselves in behaviors which are often labeled as 'ignorance' or 'communications problems'. By contrast, participation which fosters autonomous organization and self-determined activity can have a wide range of benefits besides reducing malaria. Benefits may include improved social organization, the promulgation of more scientific attitudes, and the reduction of superstitious fatalism. These can lead to other health activities, such as the promotion of breast feeding, immunization, and family planning, and promote economic activities such as the establishment of village industries, credit and agricultural cooperatives, road building, and water management.

Problems of Spraying

Spraying homes to kill mosquitoes at first seemed like the ideal method to reduce contact between humans and mosquitoes. It was simple, inexpensive, and required little health education or involvement of the local population. The original eradication program of the World Health Organization, with its uniform regulations and coordinated, routine methods for spraying throughout the country, even limited the potential for community participation. Passive acceptance of the program designed and run by others did little to promote better social organization; indeed, it may have reinforced people's feelings of helplessness and isolation. This may be why externally-run spray activities sometimes encountered apathy or outright hostility from the local people. (Barnes, 1968; Rosenfield, 1981).

A recognition of the inability to eradicate the disease by conventional methods in many areas and the subsequent reformulation of strategy to promote ongoing control efforts has led to a reevaluation of the potential contribution of communities to anti-malarial efforts. This approach demands flexibility in planning, sensitivity to local needs, and a stress on health education and motivation. The maintenance of high levels of community participation requires a high motivational level among community members. Such levels of motivation have seldom been sustained. "For example, in areas where malaria has long been endemic, it is often hard to obtain community support and acceptance, let alone participation in control programs". (Rosenfield, 1981:531). This is because the active involvement of communities for health tasks often requires a redistribution of power from government officials and local elites to here-to-fore underrepresented sectors of the population. Lacking a process of political education and organization among marginalized sectors of the society, community participation schemes may merely reinforce the power of traditional elites. (APHA, 1982).

Voluntary Collaborators

The networks of community level malaria workers and unpaid volunteers have been used in some countries for a variety of related activities, including other vector control campaigns, spraying to control other parasites, improving and monitoring local sanitation, collecting vital statistics, teaching literacy and adult education, first aid, nutrition education, and diagnostic referrals to health centers. Community run methods of malaria control can include personal protective measures, environmental engineering to control mosquito breeding sites, health education, and the diagnosis and treatment of malaria cases.

The idea of using non-salaried, volunteer collaborators to assist malaria programs in diagnosing cases and dispensing medicines originated in Latin America. As early as 1937, the malaria control program in Venezuela had organized treatment centers in post offices and schools. At present, voluntary collaborators in the villages throughout Latin America play an important role in case detection and malaria treatment. Chin reports that more than any other section of the anti-malaria program, the voluntary collaborators were responsible for the near elimination of malaria mortality in El Salvador. (Chin, 1979). In other countries of Latin America and Africa they have brought an early recognition of rising epidemics and have helped to limit the duration and severity of disease transmission.

Malaria Control in Nicaragua

Nicaragua is located in Central America, between Honduras and Costa Rica and bordering both the Atlantic and Pacific oceans. Its population of approximately three million is primarily engaged in agriculture, and more than half the people live in rural areas. Roughly a quarter of the people and most of the industry is located in the capital city, Managua. Until 1979, more than half of the population was illiterate. Nicaraguans have suffered from some of the highest mortality rates, poorest nutritional indices, and lowest levels of per capita income in the Americas [Garfield, 1984]. The biggest public health program undertaken in the 1960's and 1970's was malaria control, largely under the direction of U.S. funding organizations. Their efforts focused primarily on intra-domiciliary sprayings of DDT and related chemicals. Throughout the 20 years of malaria control efforts, short term gains from the introduction of new pesticides were wiped out by the long term resistance to the chemicals among mosquitoes. Although mortality was largely eliminated through the program, only limited progress was gained in reducing morbidity.

The incidence of malaria in Nicaragua was near an all time low in 1978 when the revolutionary war in which Sandinist overthrew the Somoza regime brought conventional malaria control activities nearly to a halt. Although the civil war ended in July 1979, it was not until 1980 that the traditional structure of spraying for malaria control was reestablished. By that time the annual parasite index had more than doubled (Halperin, 1982). Besides further developing traditional anti-malaria activities, a series of mass campaigns were utilized for malaria control. The first such activity occurred in 1980 during a national literacy campaign in which 100,000 volunteers, most of them youngsters, went to rural areas for 5 months to teach reading and writing. Eleven thousand of these literacy workers received a week of training in health matters, including malaria diagnosis and control. In July and August of 1981, clean-up campaigns were held to eliminate unhygienic conditions and mosquito breeding sites. This was followed in November of the same year with a massive campaign to administer prophylactic and curative anti-malarial medicines to the entire population of the country. Acknowledging the limits of pesticide warfare against the malaria carrying mosquito, this "final offensive" sought to use drugs to reduce the number of cases for a short period of time, reduce the transmission of the disease (by reducing the reservoir of infection in the human population) for a longer period of time, and get common people interested and involved in malaria control for an extended period of time. It was a massive undertaking, made feasible by governmental support and an effective organizational network. The drug taking campaign called for each of the 2.8 million Nicaragua citizens over one year of age to take anti-malarial medication for a consecutive three day period. Logistical requirements were such that most of Nicaragua's public organizations took part in some way. For the six weeks preceding the campaign, community groups, government workers, and school children packed over 35 million tablets into 9 million envelopes, color-coded by dosage for different age groups. The organization for young people went to work two weeks before the drug administration date taking a census and explaining to the population on a door-to-door basis the reasons for the campaign. In total, the campaign mobilized 80,000 trained volunteers and twice as many helpers, comprising a total of about 10% of the country's population. Since that November activity, ongoing campaign activities including focal reduction have been implemented.

Politicization of Nicaragua's Health Campaign

Not all were in accord with the experiment. The directors of the Nabisco factory in the capital city did not allow malaria workers to enter their plant for the census. Several priests in the north of the country told parishioners not to respond to census takers, whom they accused of spying, and to refuse the medication because they would "spread communism". The greatest resistance came from an organization of doctors and pharmacists associated with a rightist political party. They aroused fears by publicizing supposed cases of hemorrhage, birth defects, unexpected instant death and even suicide among women and children taking the anti-malarial medication. The campaign grew so politicized that the neighborhood block organization petitioned the government to oppose the plan as illegal. The government upheld the right of individual choice, but used every conceivable public forum to convince the public that it should participate. An effective network of local organization, from women's groups to peasant unions, effectively blanketed the country with pro-campaign information.

The results were impressive. More than 85% of the country's estimated population was counted in a special census for the malaria campaign. About 80% of these people took some or all of the three day drug regimen, comprising 70% of the country's population. (Garfield, 1983). Participation varied with age, state of residence, and degree of urbanization. Generally speaking, the best coverage was among young children and adults. It is presumed that older children are less concerned about their health and less easily controlled by adults than young children. Coverage varied markedly between urban and rural areas. In Masaya state, for example, coverage was 49% in the cities and close to 100% in the rural areas. This was partly related to difficulties in the census; many people were miscounted or not at home in the cities to receive the drugs. By contrast, rural residents with better community organization were known to wait for hours at the nearest road to make sure they would receive them. As a whole, states varied from a low of 29% to a high of nearly 100% in coverage of the population. A high correlation was found in interstate variations in levels of coverage for the literacy and malaria campaigns. This suggests that 37% of the differences in coverage in these campaigns relate to local organizational conditions in the states.

Routine monthly reporting data from the Nicaragua's Ministry of Health show a considerable reduction in the number of malaria cases for four months following the drug administration. Benefits of longer duration include improved community organization which permitted the rapid and efficient action to prevent destruction when much of the country was hit by floods several months later. Most Nicaraguan leaders commented at that time that they had never seen such efficient coordination and willingness to help during previous disasters.

The developments are paralleled by other recent improvements in social welfare. Infant mortality has fallen 30%, to 86 per 1000, and the literate sector of the population has risen from 48% to 88%.

Long Term Benefits

Many community organizations, especially the women's group, felt that the campaign helped them to develop leadership structures and define their role in local communities. For many women, participation in the campaigns was the first activity they engaged in outside the home. The social and political skills they developed leaves them uniquely prepared to take part in other decisions and actions in their communities along with other organizations like workers' groups, farmer organizations, student groups, and church groups.

Several of these activities relate to malaria control. Heightened awareness of malaria and its symptoms now encourage more rapid reporting and cure of cases. The traditional system of reporting posts for diagnosis and treatment in isolated areas is being further promoted. Greater local activity in malaria control is paralleled by the greater responsibility taken at the local level. Since Nicaragua's anti-malaria campaign in 1981, each local community is maintaining records of its malaria cases. This encourages local evaluation of the anti-malaria activities undertaken and may lead to better choices of the methods to use and when to use them to achieve the maximum benefit in each area.

The mass drug campaign was largely successful because it motivated a large proportion of the national population to take part in a one-time event which was low in personal risk and potentially high in health benefits. That it is the largest and most successful attempt on this scale to involve a population in collective drug taking attests to the quality of health education and the level of community organization achieved. Yet the requirements to achieve a sustained voluntary participation for on-going health activities is even greater than for this 3 day campaign. Repeated anti-malarial drug campaigns in Latin America, for example, have found decreased willingness to participate over time. Finally, it may be necessary to provide some kind of payment to volunteers in order to secure their continued participation in long term tasks.

The Nicaraguan project would not be appropriate for all malarious countries. Some nations have mosquitoes in such abundance that massive drug dosages would need to be repeated every week to eliminate the disease. As the results in Nicaragua show, mass administration of antimalarial drugs can reduce the disease for a short time, but cannot alone solve the disease problem. To provide drugs throughout a small country requires a great deal of leadership, coordination, and voluntary labor. Its long-term benefits are only likely to be realized when structures are built in communities throughout the country to involve the people in health care, as in Nicaragua.

References

American Public Health Association (1982) Primary Health Care: Progress and Problems. Washington, D.C.

Barnes, S. (1968) "Malaria Eradication in Surinam: Prospects of Success." International Journal of Health Education 1:20–31.

Bruce-Chwatt, L. S. (1980) *Essential Malariology*, William Heinemann Medical Books Ltd., London.

Chin, W. *Guidelines for Analysis of Communicable Disease* (1979) *Control* Planning, Chapter 3, Malaria, DHEW Pub. No (DHS) 79-50080.

Dunn, F. L. (1979) "Behavioral Aspects of the Control of Parasitic Diseases", W.H.O. Bulletin, 57(4):499–512.

Economic Commission for Latin America (1973) "Popular Participation in Development." Community Development Journal 2:77–92.

Farid, M. A. (1980) "The Malaria Program—From Euphoria to Anarchy". WHO Forum 1:1–10.

Garcia, G. and Najera, J. A. (1972) "The Interrelationships of Malaria, Agriculture, and the Use of Pesticides in Malaria Control". WHO Bulletin 3:15–23.

Garfield, R. and Vermund S. (1983) Changes in Malaria Incidence After a Mass Drug Administration Campaign in Managua; The Laucet, #5072, August 27, pp 500–503.

Halperin, D. and Garfield, R. (1982) "Developments in Health Care in Nicaragua". New England Journal of Medicine 307:388–392.

Harrison, G. (1978) *Mosquitoes, Malaria, and Man*, E. P. Dutton, N.Y.

Najera, J. A. (1979) "A Suggested Approach to Malaria Control". PAHO Bulletin 13:223–234.

Rosenfield, PL and Widstrand, C. G. and Ruderman, A. P. (1981) "Social and Economic Research in the UNDP/World Bank/WHO Special Program for Research and Training in Tropical Diseases". Social Science and Medicine 15A:529–538.

United States Government Accounting Office (1982) Malaria Control in Developing Countries, Washington, D.C.

Wessen, A. F. (1972) "Human Ecology and Malaria". American Journal of Tropical Medicine and Hygiene 5:658–662.

World Health Organization (1984) "Malaria Control as Part of Primary Health Care". Technical Report Series 712, Geneva.

CHAPTER 17

Health Care in a Pluralistic Society: Lebanon, Past and Present

Fuad Joseph Dagher

Despite political, religious and ethnic pluralism in Lebanon, the standard of medical education and health care were, until the first civil war in 1975, among the highest in the Arab Middle East. Nonetheless, ensuing wars have done much to erode its previously high standards. Until Lebanon ends its wars and rids itself of political extremism, health care will continue to suffer.

Introduction

WHILE MUCH HAS BEEN WRITTEN ABOUT THE POLITICAL, social, economic and administrative developments of Lebanon, little has been written about health care in this war torn country. Lebanon's large number of casualties and larger number of refugees have drastically affected health care delivery and health care priorities.

Lebanon is a small country with multiple political interest groups. There are native Lebanese which consist of diverse

Christian sects, Sunni and Shi'ite Moslems, and minority groups such as Armenians, Druze and Jews. Other groups include western missionaries who initially came to Lebanon to promote Christian education and religious conversion. Later, these missionaries played key roles in supporting and influencing education at all levels, including medical education and health care provisions. Finally, the political interest groups represent the multi-faceted ideologies and political beliefs of a number of different middle eastern countries, each promoting the objectives of their own respective nationalism. This latter group includes the Palestinians, Syrians, Iranians, Iraqis, Libyans and Israelis.

Before the war of 1975, the standard of medical education and health care in Lebanon, like the standard of literacy and education, was amongst the highest in the Arab Middle East. The most important factors for such high standards were the institutions of higher learning and their monopoly over education in the country. The American University of Beirut and the Universite Saint Joseph were the most influential in this regard and were effective in introducing western ideas and cultures to this area (Hanna, 1979). However, with the advent of war in Lebanon since 1975, the development of both medical education and health care delivery on all levels has been seriously hampered. Furthermore, Lebanon's fragmentation and warring factions have led to drastic changes in health care priorities. The objectives of primary health care and preventive medicine were displaced by the need to care for the injured and practice of therapeutic medicine.

The purpose of this chapter is to describe the sequential developments of the health care systems and health care delivery traditionally practiced in Lebanon since its independence and to ascertain the effects of the most recent events on the provision of health care and education.

Information and essential statistical data about health care in Lebanon is scarce if not unavailable. The ravaging war has made what little documentation there is almost impossible to obtain. However, when obtained, recent health data often is either fragmentary or specialized enough pertaining to a limited number of select indicators or a specific disease entity.

The Country: The People

The demographic makeup of a population is important for understanding and establishing the nature and seriousness of health problems to which it is susceptible. It is also important to determine the relationship between the economic development, the standard of living and education of the people and their needs for health care.

Lebanon is a small state on the eastern end of the Mediterranean Sea with an area of 3,950 square miles. It is bounded on the west by the Mediterranean Sea, on the north and east by Syria and on the south by Israel. In 1971, its population was estimated at 3.1 million people with an annual growth rate of 3.1 percent (Al-Any, 1981). The population density ranges between 63 per square miles, in underpopulated areas, to 1000 in the vicinity of Beirut, but averages about 780 persons per square mile. Forty-two percent of its population is urban.

Historically, Lebanon was formed from five adjacent districts within the Turkish or Ottoman Empire. Under Greek, Roman, Arab and Ottoman domination, this area of the Middle East was a trading center and a refuge for religious minorities, mainly Christians, but also included Moslems, Druze and Jews. In 1920 after the first world war, Lebanon became an independent state and was placed under the French mandate between 1920 and 1941. In 1946 French troops withdrew and Lebanon was granted its full independence.

Topographically, the country may be divided into four main areas: A narrow coastal plain, a coastal mountain range extending from the Cedars of Lebanon in the north rising to as high as 10,115 feet to Mount Hermon in the south, a narrow central valley, the Biqa' Valley plateau east to the coastal mountains and the interior mountain range, the anti-Lebanon range, bordering Syria with elevations up to 9,055 feet.

Arabic is the official national language as well as the religious language of the Moslem and the Druze communities.
French is the second language for most educated people while
English is also widely spoken. Armenian is spoken and taught
among the Armenian population.

The political climate of Lebanon consists of mosaic religious
communities which, in one way or another, influence medical
education and health care. Although the government main-
tains a population register, it has not carried out a popular
census since 1932. Registration is usually incomplete and
accurate figures for Lebanese nationals and religious communities are not well known. The problem has been further
compounded by the influx of thousands of non-Lebanese al-
iens moving into the country, as well as by forced re-distribu-
tion of large segments of the Lebanese population resulting
from ongoing wars and invasions. The Moslems, both Shi'ites
and Sunnis, presently constitute the majority of the Lebanese
population, with the Shi'ites taking the lead. Next in number
are the Christians. In this group, the Maronites are the majority. The Maronites trace their origin to Saint Maron, a Syrian
hermit monk of the late fourth and early fifth century who
founded the Maronite church. In the middle of the sixth and
early seventh century, large numbers of his followers moved
to the rugged mountains of northern Lebanon. Other Christians include Roman Catholics, Greek Catholics, Greek Orthodox, Armenian Catholics, Nestorians, Armenian Orthodox
and Protestants. Still other religious minorities include
Druzes, Jews, Bahais, and Seventh Day Adventists.

Foreign influence has been very strong. Missionaries from
France, the United States, Britain and Russia have been
active since the 19th Century. They have not, however, been
very successful in converting Moslems and other non-Chris-
tians to Christianity, but were most successful in converting
Christians from one church or one sect to another. Each of
these missionaries developed and supported educational systems similar to the ones in their own countries. However,
varying degrees of modifications by private and parochial

schools were instituted by Christians as well as Moslem religious communities. Such influences led to the spread of organizational complexes and culturally diverse educational systems which resulted in the high rate of education (86%) in Lebanon, the highest among the Arab Middle East.

Medical and Health Problems

Education is highly valued in Lebanon. There are five universities in Beirut alone. These include the American University, the French Jesuit University (Universite Saint Joseph), the Beirut University College, the Lebanese State University and the Beirut Arab University. Others include the National Academy of Arts plus a number of smaller colleges and institutions. In addition, thousands of Lebanese go abroad for their higher or post-doctorate education and over thirty thousand foreigners come to study in Lebanon every year. The first two institutions, the American University and Universite Saint Joseph, the oldest in the country, have health science schools including schools of medicine, hygiene and preventive medicine, nursing and dental schools.

According to Webster's New World Dictionary, pluralism is defined as: a) "the existence within a nation or society of groups distinctive in ethnic origin, cultural habits, religion or the like," and b) "a policy favoring the preservation of such groups within a given nation or society." Lebanon as an independent sovereign country perfectly exemplifies the definition of pluralism. While it is a democratic state since it became independent in 1947, Lebanon has continued to exist as a democracy while preserving the pluralistic nature of its populace and simultaneously trying to preserve the Arabism of Lebanon. The responsible sequential governments of the country throughout the years since independence tried (though not successfully) to implement and institute new projects in health care. Unfortunately, early on following the second world war, intentionally or otherwise, health care was not considered a major priority. In addition, the fragmented political system in Lebanon led to a weak central government that both encouraged and tolerated factionalism. There was reliance on private militia even before the civil war. The central government had little power and consequently had limited social and health services as well as little aid for further development.

Nevertheless, there were adequate provisions for hygiene and basic health care in the capital city of Beirut and perhaps in a few other large cities. In contrast, the rural areas of the south, north and interior Lebanon, the Biqa' Valley and Ba'albeck exemplified only poor health services. Health care provision was mainly provided by a few private charitable and religious organizations supported by private money. The government provided clinics and dispensaries, albeit few, but these were poorly equipped, poorly stocked and often times inadequately staffed with part-time employees and physicians.

With time, help and assistance from experts in the fields of medicine and health care from the two main institutions of higher education in Lebanon, and with additional help from international world organizations such as The World Health Organization (WHO) and United Nations Education and Scientific Organization (UNESCO), the government began to address the issue of health in a more scientific and industrialized fashion. They looked at health not only as lack of disease, but as maximum personal comfort, i.e., physical, social and emotional. When governmental agencies started addressing health care, health education and hygiene in schools, the concept of primary care, family medicine, preventive medicine, maternal and child health, provision of basic medicine and immunization and vaccination were conceived. With this approach, the emphasis began to shift from that of primarily therapeutic medicine to preventive medicine. Government sponsored hospitals, clinics and dispensaries mushroomed throughout the country. While these projects were mostly government supported and sponsored, health insurance as known in the West was non-existent.

People who did not want to seek care in government sponsored clinics and hospitals sought assistance and care at private clinics and private hospitals, thus paying for these services from their own private sources. In 1964 the government instituted a social security system with a medical service plan. However, this scheme was available only to civil service employees and their families as well as large employers who partly contributed to the insurance coverage of their employees. In addition to the social security medical service plan, other insurance plans were provided by the civil servant unions, the medical establishments of the armed forces and the internal security and by support from the ministry of health. The latter either built new government hospitals or contracted with private hospitals for beds to take care of a certain defined number of people. By so doing, the government directly or indirectly was able to insure health care for just under 2 million of its population or 68% of the Lebanese population. The remaining populace was covered by some type of private insurance or charitable organizations such as the Red Cross and the Red Crescent organizations. As a direct result of these health care provisions, infant mortality decreased significantly and longevity of life increased (Azar, 1982). The death rate decreased to around 9 per 1000 while child birth increased 34 per 1000, resulting in a growth rate of over 20 per 1000. Furthermore, because of the prospering economy and a better, more comfortable life in Lebanon, specialists and well-trained physicians and surgeons were returning to the country after spending several years of postdoctoral education and training in such countries as the United States, France, Germany, England, Russia and the Eastern European block. In the early 1970's the economy of Lebanon boomed as evidenced by the large numbers of foreign banking institutions in Beirut. More attention was given to health care, and in the field of medicine, superspecialization became evident. As a result, several advances in medicine and surgery were achieved; for example, Lebanon was the first country in the Arab Middle East to perform open heart surgery and kidney transplantation operations on patients.

The War and Its Effects

During Lebanon's period of prosperity in the 1970's, political factionalism existing in the country blocked the establishment of national identity that might have helped to bring together this fragmented society. Furthermore, Lebanon's problems which are its own, have been compounded by the existing Israeli, Palestinian, Syrian and Jordanian conflicts. In 1948 tens of thousands of Palestinians fleeing northern Palestine made their way across the border into southern Lebanon; by 1952 they numbered over 150,000 people. Since they were largely Moslems, they posed a special problem for Lebanon's very delicate political balance. With the 1967 war, a new influx of Palestinian refugees from the West Bank of Palestine came to Lebanon and between 1970 and 1971, after Jordan's King Hussein's armies drove out Palestinian guerillas from that country, most of the fighters and their families ended up in Lebanon. The weak Lebanese government and army could not suppress the Palestinian forces who had significant support from sectors of the Lebanese public. By the mid 1970's, the Palestinian population had grown to over 300,000 or 10% of the Lebanese population. They could not possibly be assimilated. They were supported by most Muslims in Lebanon and by a few liberal and left wing Christian Lebanese. Palestinian attacks against Israel continued and caused the latter to intervene in Lebanon with tremendous force thus exacerbating sectarian tensions. The Palestinians were living together in full communities with a governing structure of their own, with social and health services and substantial armed forces; they became a state within a state.

Under this scenario, the civil war started in 1975 and with it, every governmental and private project, including health projects, came to a standstill and an enormous number of problems erupted. By the time this first Lebanese civil war came to an end in 1976, the human toll and suffering had been staggering. Over 65,000 men, women and children were killed (AFSC, 1982). Some 1.5 million people were uprooted from their homes in cities and villages and more than 400,000 had been victims of the war as wounded, displaced, abandoned or orphaned, all in a country of 3 million people. With Lebanon's infrastructure destroyed, so was the water supply, sewers, roads and public utilities. There was lack of sanitation and hygiene, and public health problems became enormous. Epidemics of typhoid fever, dysentery, encephalitis and even poliomyelitis erupted. Because of crowding and poor hygiene, even pulmonary tuberculosis and typhus began to appear among Lebanese and Palestinian refugees. During the civil war of 1975–76, social and government institutions hardly functioned and when they did, they did so at a marginal level. Health care was mainly limited to treating casualties if these could be brought to hospitals. Hospitals which remained functional were crowded. For example, one such hospital, the American University Hospital in Beirut, treated 10,000 casualties between 1975 and 1976 despite shortages in medical supplies and in medical and para-medical nursing staff (Asper, 1978), (Shehadeh, 1977). The war was finally brought to a halt through the introduction of 30,000 Syrian troops who have since remained. Their continued presence raises the question of their long-term intentions.

From then on Lebanon continued to be a battle field for feuding middle eastern countries. As though Lebanon has not suffered enough through its civil war, it was further violated by being cast directly into the middle of the Israeli/Palestinian conflict. With that, health care, among many other vital issues, continued to suffer and deteriorate. The Israelis stepped up attacks against Palestinian refugee camps, villages and military installations in southern Lebanon where Palestinian groups staged repeated attacks on Israeli territories. The victims of such attacks were not Palestinian fighters, but Palestinian and Lebanese civilians. In 1978, a full scale Israeli

assault and invasion into Lebanon resulted in 200,000
Lebanese and 65,000 Palestinian refugees fleeing the area.
These homeless people were relocated in the suburbs of
Beirut, thus compounding the already poor medical and public health conditions existing at the time. The political and
military situation continued in turmoil until things came to a
head by the Israeli invasion and occupation of the southern
part of Lebanon in 1982, which resulted in the expulsion of
the Palestinian fighters by Israelis from Beirut and, at a later
date, their expulsion from Tripoli by the Syrians. As a direct
result, more casualties, more refugees and, more repatriation
of these refugees created additional health hazards.

New bouts of fighting once again led to hundreds of thousands of new refugees being forced to move into new areas
which were neither prepared nor equipped to receive them,
creating additional burdens to local governments and further
compounding the public health problems. A census was conducted by the Catholic Center for Information in three
Lebanese counties in the mountain regions east of Beirut
involving 111 villages and towns (Rahmi, 1983). As seen in
Table 1, there was a total of 206,384 people in these counties.
Between August 31, 1983 and October 6, 1983, 59.37 percent
or 122,523 people were forced to leave their homes and flee to
other locations while 1,363 people died or disappeared.

With the country partitioned and the war continuing una-
bated, primary health care was once again non-existent in
Lebanon. Most medicine and health care was catered to the
casualties of the war. Once again, medical care became dependent on the private sector with no significant coordination
between the private and the governmental health sector.
While in the 1970's for every dollar spent on preventive medicine, 22 dollars were spent for therapeutic medicine, in 1982
for every dollar spent on public health medicine, 128 dollars
were spent on therapeutic care. A large portion of these
expenses were and continued to be paid by the citizens themselves. Over 6 percent of peoples' incomes covered medical

Table 1

Casualties (Fleeing and Dead People) in Three Counties
in the Mountains East of Beirut, Between August 31, 1983
and October 6, 1983.

Counties	Number of People	Number of People Forced to Flee		Dead
Ba'Bda	19914	16649	(83.81%)	122
Shouf Mountains	75464	39154	(51.88%)	544
Aley	111006	66720	(60.11%)	697
TOTAL	206384	122523	(59.37%)	1263

care and the cost of drugs; the fourth major expense after food, education and housing compared to only 3 percent in France.

The wars in Lebanon have disrupted the country's health care delivery system and created a great need for preventative and environmental health care services. Instead of asking government authorities for elementary public health guarantees, the Lebanese citizen would prefer that the government would provide safety for him and for his family. He cannot demand health care for himself and for his family when their very existence is in danger. Furthermore, who is he to ask or demand from, a government which itself is threatened and pre-occupied with various problems and emergencies or his employer who too may be threatened with destruction and bankruptcy? Under these circumstances, the Lebanese remain quite content with buying medical therapy and medicine the way they buy bread and food for their families.

Health care services in the area of preventative care are nearly non-existent. Nevertheless the government attempts to offer therapeutic medical services as it can. To illustrate this policy, as recent as January, 1984, the government has contracted with 84 (54 percent of the total) of 124 private hospitals in Lebanon to insure the availability of 1180 additional beds for the treatment of casualties of the war. Presently in Lebanon, there are approximately 8000 hospital beds while the recommended number of hospital beds for countries with a population equal to that of Lebanon is 12,000 beds. Four thousand additional beds are, therefore, badly needed, even without considering the altered demographic status of the country.

In its constitution and bylaws, the World Health Organization refers to "Health" as not only a lack of disease, but as maximum personal comfort, and physical, social and emotional well-being. Until Lebanon ends its wars, rids itself of its extreme political pluralistic tendencies as well as its deep ideological divisions between its different religious, ethnic and socioeconomic groups, "HEALTH" will remain a far fetched objective.

References

Al-Any, Nancy W., et al. (1984) Area Handbook for Lebanon. Harvey H. Smith, New York.

Azar, Joseph (1982) "Health and the Number of Hospital Beds in the Year 2000." Al-Nahar Daily Newspaper, Beirut, Lebanon, April 23.

American Friends Service Committee (AFSC): (1982) A Compassionate Peace: A Future for the Middle East. Hill and Wang, New York.

Asper, Samuel (1978) "An American in Beirut." Bulletin of the American College of Surgeons 63:5–10.

Hanna, Faith M. (1979) An American Mission: The Role of the American University of Beirut, Boston, Alphabet Press.

Rahmi, George (Father) (1983) Daily News Agency—Lebanon Census of the Catholic Center for Information.

Shehadeh, Sameer (1977) "Anatomy of a Hospital in Distress." Bulletin of the American College of Surgeons 62:6–7.

CHAPTER 18

Policy for Primary Health Care in Lebanon

Rashid Bashshur, Nabil Kronfol, and Elizabeth Aby Haydar

Discussed are the comprehensive health policy developed
in Lebanon in the shadows of civil war and foreign occupation, that asserts the rights of all citizens to good health. Its
cornerstone is the Area Health Authority, a regional model
for the organization, co-ordination, and finance of the delivery of health and social services.

Introduction

VIOLENCE IN LEBANON HAS ATTRACTED WORLDWIDE AT-
tention for nearly a decade. This small country of about 2.6
million people and a land area of around 10,000 square kilometers has experienced a protracted civil war between political and religious factions, strongly fueled by outside forces. In
addition, Lebanon has witnessed the occupation of most of its
land area by outside armies. Nonetheless, when given real-
istic chances for taking control of its own affairs, free of outside
influence, Lebanon has shown strong signs of resilience and
vitality. One such example is the development of a new com-

prehensive health policy, to meet the health needs of the people through efficient and effective regional programs with emphasis on primary care, disease prevention and health promotion. This national policy is part of a large scale effort undertaken by the Government of Lebanon to reunite its people and to reform and modernize its health care institutions. Planning for this policy began in 1980, and was ratified by the new government in 1986. Its formal enactment into law occurred in several stages, culminating with the full reorganization of the Ministry of Health and Social Affairs.

Historical Background of Public Health System

Lebanon was proclaimed an independent country in 1943, after an agreement was reached between a provisional government in exile and French authorities to end 25 years of the French Mandate which extended over the area that now comprises both Syria and Lebanon. Although the French may have preferred to stay longer, they were not pushed out of Lebanon by force. They left behind their brand of cumbersome bureaucracy and a civil service that was predominantly trained by the French. This included the Ministry of Public Health (MOPH), the laws that govern its functions and operations and, at least initially, several of its key administrative personnel. The role of the MOPH was purposefully restricted to *public health* activities, as defined at that time, namely to protect the health of the *public* from the spread of epidemics, infectious diseases and pests and to provide medical services to the poor and destitute through government facilities. Thus, it was barred from any significant involvement in the delivery or regulation of medical services.

Since Lebanon's independence from the French in 1943 to the present time, there have been several attempts on the part of the Government of Lebanon to expand the scope of the Ministry of Public Health and to introduce health and welfare programs. The two most notable of these programs are the

National Social Security Fund (NSSF), a national insurance scheme, and the Office of Social Development (OSD), a regional program for organizing and coordinating social, educational and health services. The national insurance scheme (NSSF) incorporated three separate funds: (1) the retirement and end-of-service benefits to government employees, (2) old age benefits, and (3) sickness and maternity benefits. The Office of Social Development, (OSD), created in 1959 as an autonomous board within the Ministry of Labor and Social Affairs, was charged with responsibility for developing programs in health, education, social welfare, and community development. In contrast to the National Social Security Fund (NSSF), the OSD had very strong ties to the private sector, and it subsidized private charitable organizations, both religious and secular, as well as community based art, crafts and folklore projects. However, rather than being incorporated into the Ministry of Public Health, these two programs were established as separate, autonomous agencies with very weak and ineffective links to Lebanon's health Ministry.

Another example of the fragmentary uncoordinated approach that characterized previous efforts to introduce health care reform is the regulation of hospitals. When the Ministry of Public Health tried to introduce regulations over hospitals dealing with quality and cost control, they created instead another semi-autonomous national agency, the National Hospital Board. This Board never concerned itself with regulating hospitals. Instead, it served more as a trade association than a regulatory agency whose primary objective was the protection of the interests of its constituents.

Consistent with Lebanon's free enterprise system, the private sector in medicine has been traditionally strong. The civil war made it even stronger because of the breakdown of public authority and the need for medical personnel and facilities available mostly in the private sector. The few operating government facilities, such as hospitals and dispensaries, were inadequately staffed and ineffective in meeting the demand for patients who were subsidized by the Government.

The Ministry of Public Health has 12 general hospitals and a total capacity of 1543 beds. However, these numbers fluctuated during the past decade with the level of hostilities in the different areas of the country. For example, a survey conducted in 1982 revealed that only 573 of these beds were operational (Kronfol, 1982). In contrast, there were 18 private not-for-profit hospitals with a total bed capacity of 3219 and 68 for-profit hospitals with a bed capacity of 3390. Of the total bed capacity of 6609 available in the private sector, 5714 were found operational in 1982. In addition, the average occupancy rate in the private hospitals was about 60 percent whereas it was only about 50 percent in public hospitals. Hence, the toll of the war has been much more devastating on the public sector as compared to the private. More importantly, however, the Ministry of Public Health was contributing about 68 percent of its budget to these private hospitals (Jeffers and Zukin, 1982).

In brief, the conclusion reached by the special Health Assessment and Planning Mission of the World Health Organization and the League of Red Cross and Red Crescent Societies (WHO/LRCS) is a fair statement regarding the condition of the Ministry in 1983. ". . . the organization, financing and delivery of health services are fragmented and chaotic. . . The Ministry of Public Health (MOPH) sees two-thirds of its budget paid to the private sector as uncontrolled reimbursement for private hospital services of uncertain quality and necessity. . ." (WHO/LRCS, 1983:7).

The Genesis of the New Health Policy

The first efforts at planning for primary health care were initiated in 1980 during the height of the civil war by a local community in Lebanon, represented by the Council of Municipalities of the Upper Metn region. This local community represented a mix of Lebanon's population in terms of its religious composition, though it tended to be predominantly middle class. Its Council requested technical assistance in the development of an optimal health system model that could be tested initially in their community and eventually disseminated throughout the country (AUB, 1980). The model was revived within a broader comprehensive health policy by the Government that assumed office in 1982 during a period of relative stability, from November 1982 to September 1983. During this time a new President of the Republic was unanimously elected by the Parliament, and an era of optimism prevailed. It was widely hoped that a permanent settlement would be reached between the warring factions and that foreign occupation forces would leave. The new government reinforced these views.

During this period, the cabinet was granted extraordinary (but temporary) powers by the Parliament to enact new legislation, particularly in the areas of reconstruction and consolidation, with emphasis on health, housing, and economic development. The Ministry of Public Health (MOPH) capitalized on the temporary powers and introduced massive legislation reforms that not only consolidated most health agencies at the new Ministry of Health and Social Affairs, but also embarked on a comprehensive regional program based on the precepts of primary health care and regionalization.

When considered in the broader context of the condition of a country emerging from a civil war, the activities of the Ministry in this regard are significant in at least two different respects: (1) The extensive planning and developmental activities have demonstrated the serious commitment of the Government of Lebanon to large-scale health care reform. (2) The coalescence of various viewpoints and factions around health care issues demonstrated how concerted work in health affairs can yield fruitful results. The planning and legislative activities served as a catalyst that brought together people with divergent convictions and viewpoints. Thus, it may be argued that if the warring factions can be involved in joint health planning and the development of joint health programs, as well as in other areas of mutual vital interest then the level of hostility between them would subside. Perhaps too much can be made of this point, but in view of the self-destructive course in which the country is headed any positive indicator of progress toward reconciliation should be noted and emphasized.

Preparation for New Policy

The preparation for the development of the new health policy was quite extensive, and it included the use of national and international resources. It included the following major activities:

(a) The Minister requested a comprehensive self study of the Ministry of Public Health for the purpose of generating proposals for change from within the Ministry. Thus, the various department and division heads were asked to conduct a self study and to submit specific recommendations for changing the laws that govern their units.

(b) Several task forces consisting of Lebanese experts in the various health fields (public health, medicine and pharmacy) were appointed without regard to their political affiliation. They were asked to review current practices at the Ministry and make specific recommendations for changes in their respective areas. These task forces included primary care, health information and statistics, pharmacy practice and drugs, environmental health, and disease surveillance and control.

(c) The World Health Organization and the International League of Red Cross and Crescent Societies (WHO/LRCS) delegated a team of international experts to conduct an on-site investigation and report their findings and recommendations. After considerable data collection and analysis, this commission submitted a detailed status report, together with a list of recommendations, specific actions and target dates for a total health system and social welfare reform (WHO/LRCS, 1983).

(d) An economic study of the financing of health care in Lebanon was undertaken under the sponsorship of the United

States Agency for International Development (USAID). A detailed analysis concerning health sector financing in Lebanon was completed together with a set of recommendations. (Jeffers and Zukin, 1983).

(e) A comprehensive plan for organizing health services in the Greater Beirut area was developed with USAID support for consideration by the World Bank as part of its aid program for the reconstruction of Lebanon. It called for the implementation of the Area Health Authority concept in the Capital. This concept will be described later in this chapter.

(f) A regional plan for the Province of South Lebanon was prepared by a British consultant group under a grant from the European Economic Community (EEC). This plan was also based on the concept of the Area Health Authority (AHA). A demonstration project was initially funded by the EEC for the establishment of a model AHA program in Southern Lebanon (Tibbald Partnership Limited, 1983).

(g) The Middle East Council of Churches, a branch of the World Council of Churches, established a model community health program in Hirmel, a remote area of Lebanon whose inhabitants are mostly Shiite Moslems. The Council had a dual purpose. The first was to provide immediate emergency medical relief and primary care to the residents of this medically underserved areas. The second and more important purpose was to support governmental efforts in developing and implementing the health policy by providing a viable demonstration site for a pilot health system.

Coming from mostly foreign and knowledgeable sources, these reports confirmed the need for reform and gave greater legitimacy to the government's efforts in this regard. Problems identified by these reviews are those of fragmentation and overlapping of private and public health care delivery, and the immense power and unaccountability of the private sector. Likewise, bureaucratic structural inefficiencies within the Ministry and competition between health and welfare agencies, combined with problems of unequal health resources and inadequate cost and quality controls created a situation desperately requiring reforms. Upon the review of these reports which provided the necessary documentation for needed changes, the Ministry commissioned the senior advisor to the Minister, a consultant to the Ministry, and two government officials to write the new laws for the reorganization of the Ministry of Health and Social Affairs, which were adopted in September 1983. The enactment of these laws is likely to have permanent effects on the health care system of Lebanon. Since these constitute the laws of the land any future government will have to reckon with them. Even if their implementation is incomplete or delayed, they can not be ignored, unless they are changed.

A major tenet of the new health and social affairs policy of Lebanon, as embodied in the new laws, is the universal entitlement of all citizens to good health and well-being and, therefore, to the receipt of the services pursuant thereof (Mroueh, 1982). This policy affirms the responsibility of the government for promoting the health and well-being of the people of Lebanon and the development of an effective partnership between the private and public sectors as well as the emphasis on individual responsibility for health. Thus, in view of the expanded role and extended responsibility of the Government in health and social affairs and the attendant costs that will be incurred in securing and providing the requisite health services to the people, it is incumbent upon the Government to design and develop a cost effective, efficient, productive and acceptable health care delivery system. The main feature of this system is the Area Health Authority, (AHA) to be described in the remainder of this chapter.

The reorganized Ministry of Health and Social Affairs will consist of two levels, (a) the central level which is responsible for national health policy, national planning, quality control, financing, regulation, evaluation and development, and (b) the local community level where the services are actually delivered to the people.

The Area Health Authority

The new health and social affairs policy encompasses a wide range of reforms in existing structures and arrangements in the public sector, the expansion of regulation over the performance and quality of the services available in both public and private sectors, and the introduction of innovative systems for the delivery of comprehensive primary health care and social services at the local community level. Its cornerstone is the Area Health Authority (AHA), a model for the organization, coordination, control and delivery of comprehensive health services, both personal and non-personal, at the community level. The model is based on the following principles:

1. *The regionalization of health services:* This entails the establishment of a hierarchy of services on the basis of the health needs of the population by geographic area.
2. *Community control:* The governance of the AHA is delegated to the local community and includes the clients and the providers of care. While responsibility to conform with national regulations is maintained, the local communities are given substantial freedom in setting up the programs most suitable to their needs and wishes.
3. *Coordination between the public and private sectors:* The AHA does not aim to supplant or replace the private practice of medicine. It does aim, however, to enhance the quality and effectiveness of health care resources available in the private sector by establishing standards of performance, by providing incentives for physicians to locate in underserved areas and by increasing the cooperation between the private and public sectors.
4. *The provision of comprehensive health services:* There is a need to coordinate and integrate all primary care activities in the service area of Lebanon's Area Health Authority, and to establish a referral network for tertiary

care inside and outside the area. This is necessary in order to avoid unnecessary overlap and duplication of services, and to create greater efficiency in the system of health care, as well as to fill in gaps that may exist.

The emphasis on prevention and health promotion is crucial. It is recognized that the health of a population is the result of several factors, including the condition of the environment, certain aspects of life style and individual behavior, genetics, and of course, medical care. Hence, the approach to be adopted by the AHA for improving the health of its service population will take into account all major factors that affect health.

The Functions of the Area Health Authority

The functions to be served by the AHA at the regional level are as follows:

(1) *Plan Development and Strategic Planning:* The first task of the AHA is the development of a comprehensive health plan for meeting the health needs of the people in its service area according to the requirements and guidelines issued by the Ministry. The designation of the service area and its population will be made by the Ministry, and it consists of a geographic area having a population between 200,000 and 300,000 with boundaries coterminous with those of civil subdivisions, such as the Qaza.

(2) *Community Health Center:* Upon approval of its plan, the AHA will be responsible for establishing a Community Health Center (CHC) for the provision, coordination and integration of the direct delivery of all health services and social services that fall under its purview. Thus, the CHC will serve as the major service unit of the AHA in each region. The type and scope of services provided by the CHC will be described under "Operations" below.

(3) **Program Management:** The Area Health Authority (AHA) will assume responsibility for the management of all programs and activities that fall under its purview. This will include the recruitment and, where indicated, the training of an administrative staff, the development of an efficient system of management with allocation of function and responsibility, and the financial management of funds in the AHA.

(5) **Monitoring and Control:** The AHA will be responsible for monitoring the cost, quality, accessibility and acceptability of care rendered either through its own facilities as well as those in the private sector who are reimbursed from public funds. These activities will be conducted in accordance with standards, criteria and procedures established by the Ministry.

(6) **Coordination and Referral:** The AHA will attempt to coordinate and integrate all the health services provided in the public and private sectors in order to minimize unnecessary and inappropriate redundancies and to promote efficiency and productivity. It will also establish a referral service to specialists and tertiary care medical centers both within and outside its service area.

Governance and Organizational Structure

The AHA shall operate under a local authority to be established by the local municipality, a council of municipalities, or other appropriate regional authority. It shall be governed by an Executive Board, an Executive Director, and an Advisory Board.

The Executive Board shall have the responsibility for establishing the basic policies of the AHA and for implementation of the national health policy established by the Ministry of Health and Social Affairs. It shall have final authority for all financial and administrative matters related to local AHA operations.

The Advisory Board shall have broad citizen participation from the entire service area of the Area Health Authority

(AHA). Its primary function is to advise the Executive Director in various matters related to Community Health Center operations and the various services rendered in the community.

The Executive Director shall be responsible for the routine managerial and administrative functions of the AHA, for executing the policies of the Executive Board, for compliance with national policies and regulations, and for the overall supervision of the Community Health Center.

Operations

The AHA will ensure that the full range of routine therapeutic personal health services (primary health care) and preventive personal health services as well as a broad range of public health activities and social services are made available to the residents of the community. Its operations are herein described in terms of the (1) services to be provided, (2) the population to be served, (3) the providers of service, and (4) the method of payment for the services.

The Services to be provided by the AHA through its own facilities and in conjunction with local medical providers will include primary health care and hospitalization for routine acute care and public health and social services. Therefore, these services are essentially limited to primary health care including prevention and public health. In addition, it will have a referral service to specialists and to tertiary care medical centers.

The Service Population of each AHA will be defined as the permanent residents who live in the designated service area. Specific boundaries for the service area will be established, and these boundaries will correspond with those of civil subdivisions in order that an entire municipality of Qaza is included.

The Providers of Service in each AHA will consist of the physicians, nurses, public health workers and other clinical and outreach personnel. All public health workers and clinical personnel, other than the doctors, will be hired by the AHA as regular employees. Physicians will be able to participate in the AHA on one of the following bases:

(a) As salaried full-time employees, or

(b) as a group medical practice who will enter into a contractual relationship with the AHA to provide services to a defined population on the basis of capitation.

In the case of salaried employment, special incentive mechanisms will be created to encourage productivity and efficiency of physicians. These incentives will be based on individual and/or group performance in terms of number of patients served, the quality of the care rendered, and overall contribution to the productivity of the Center as a whole.

A prepaid group practice contract will be negotiated with groups of physicians who organize themselves into a group practice and are willing to assume direct responsibility for providing ambulatory care and preventive services to a defined service population on a capitation basis, to be negotiated annually. Referral to specialists will be reimbursed according to a fee schedule that is agreed upon in advance with the participating physicians.

Method of Payment

For purposes of payment, the services to be provided by the AHA can be classified into two types: (a) public health and social services and (b) all other services. Public health and social services are paid from public funds and require no reimbursement.

Therapeutic and preventive services rendered to individuals, outside of the public health domain, will be subject to payment by the patient or a third party. Payments can be made in one of two ways: (a) prepayment, either directly by the individual subscriber, his or her employer, a union or other organized group, or social security. (b) The other payment method is fee-for-service and it will be based on a fee schedule. The poor and indigent will be covered by the public treasury. Arrangements will be worked out for deductibles and copayment in order to discourage unnecessary use of service.

Conclusion

The above plan has been adopted by the Government of Lebanon as a basic cornerstone of its new health policy. Funds for a large-scale demonstration of a pilot Area Health Authority in the southern suburbs of Beirut were made available from the United Nations, the United States and Italy as well as the local treasury.

Since the enactment of the new plan for primary health care, another major outbreak of violence brought about the resignation of the government that developed this plan. The new government, the Government of National Reconciliation, in reviewing legislation developed and enacted by its predecessor, singled out the above described health plan for its approval and ratification (Mroueh & Kronfol, 1986).

References

American University of Beirut, (1982) The Upper Metn Health System: A Project Proposal, Proposal Prepared by American University of Beirut, Faculty of Health Services. Beirut, Lebanon.

Jeffers, James and Paul Zukin, (1983) Lebanon Health Sector Financing: Issues, Problems and Recommendations. Report supported by the U.S. Agency for International Development, Beirut, Lebanon.

Kronfol, Nabil, (1982) Survey of Health Facilities in Lebanon, Unpublished Report, Beirut, Lebanon.

Mroueh, Adnan (1982), The Health Care System of Lebanon, A Past, A Present, and A Future, Paper Presented at the National Council on International Health, Dec. 1982, Washington, D.C.

Mroueh, Adnan and Nabil Kronfol (1986) Health Services in Lebanon, World Health Organization. Regional Office for the Eastern Mediterranean, Alexandria, Egypt. Vol. 1, 2, and 3.

Tibbald Partnership Limited, (1983) Health Planning for South Lebanon, Progress Report Financed by the European Economic Community, London.

World Health Organization, (1983) Reconstruction of the Health Services of Lebanon, Report of the WHO/LRCS Health Assessment and Planning Mission, Geneva, Switzerland.